MINDING

CORONA

2020-2022

Is Your Mind More Powerful Than the Virus?

Dr. Jean-Luc Mommaerts

M.D., M.A.I., Ph.D.

Published by AURELIS Ed. Antwerp, Belgium

www.aurelis.org

2020-2022 © Jean-Luc Mommaerts

Line-edited by Kit Duncan

April 7, 2022

MINDING CORONA: Is Your Mind More Powerful Than the Virus?

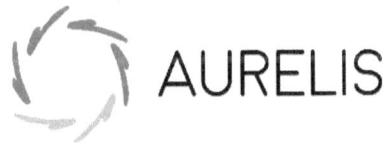

Disclaimer

The information provided in or through this book and the AURELIS websites is for educational and informational purposes only. It should not be seen as a replacement for any medical service or procedure. AURELIS is mental hygiene. There is no guarantee of accuracy and completeness of any information provided. You should not rely on this as a substitute for, nor does it replace proper professional medical advice, diagnosis or treatment. We accept no responsibility for any damage or injury. If in doubt, you should consult your physician, especially in case of a history of mental problems.

Health care providers should exercise their own independent clinical judgment when using this information or the mentioned mobile app in conjunction with patient care.

Nothing worse than a false sense of security. Please, take every measure of precaution. Then, read on.

If you are searching for the 'AURELIS Acute Stress app,' you can download it for free. Please go to the appendix *An app to support*. Or you can go to

https://aurelis.org/aurelis-app

On that same page, you find an intro video of the app.

You also find it on the app stores of Google and Apple.

To Mari

"It is much more important to know what sort of a patient has a disease than what sort of a disease a patient has." [Sir William Osler, 1849-1919, often called the Father of Modern Medicine]

Table of Contents

INTRODUCTION 11

MINDING CORONA – 12 POINTS 15

1. PANDEMIA OR GLOBAL HYSTERIA? 19

2. MIND AND CORONA 30

3. THE MESSAGE IN THE VIRUS........................... 41

4. COVID AND ATTENTION 50

5. WHAT TO DO IN TIMES OF COVID.................... 55

6. RETHINKING COVID – IN THE FACE OF STRESS 61

7. CORONA CRASH... 66

8. COVID WHIRLPOOL 71

9. WORST CASE COVID....................................... 76

10. CORONA RISK 83

11. SUMMER OF COVID 92

12. WHERE OH WHERE IS THE VIRUS IN EUROPE? 113

13. WINTER OF COVID 118

14. MOTIVATION WITHOUT ANXIETY IN CORONA TIMES....... 126

15. MIND THE DENIAL.. 135

16. POSTCORONALIA – COVID COMPLICATIONS 144

17. LEADERSHIP IN CORONA TIMES 150

18. CORONA: SUPER-STRESS, SUPER-SPREADING? 157

19. THE VIRUS IS NOT THE ENEMY 161

20. AUTUMN OF COVID: DISASTER^2 ALREADY? 169

21. HOW TO MAKE SOMEONE TAKE HIS VACCINATION 176

22. ONLY 'CONTROL' + COVID-WHIRLPOOL = DISASTER 182

23. THE FINAL COVID QUESTION: ETHICS OR ECONOMICS? ... 188

24. COVID + SCHOOL + CHILDREN 192

25. COVID COMPASSION 202

26. MINDING CORONA, SAVING LIVELIHOODS AND LIVES 208

27. THE PROBLEM WITH CORONA IS THE PROBLEM WITH MEDICINE 215

28. MOTIVATING CROWDS IN CORONA TIMES 220

29. OUR MIND IS OUR WAY OUT (OR INTO) COVID 227

30. COVID: WHY HIDING THE MIND? 234

31. COVID MANAGEMENT AT SOCIETY LEVEL 238

32. COVID: STILL FLYING ON ONE WING 247

33. CAN MIND ACUTELY PREVENT COVID? 252

34. MILLIONS OF UNNEEDED COVID DEATHS IN 2021? 260

35. VACCINATION HESITANCY: THE GOOD, THE LESS GOOD, AND THE UGLY 266

36. VACCINE OR VACCINATION? 274

37. 1.5 YEARS OF MINDLESS COVID 283

38. WINTER OF 2021: COVID WINTER AGAIN!? 290

39. WHAT IF COVID VACCINATIONS ARE 80% PLACEBO? 293

40. PROVING AND USING THE MIND IN COVID 302

41. NO PSYCHE IN COVID? — OR NO COVID WITHOUT PSYCHE?
.... 309

42. NOT YET OUT OF THE WOODS! 315

43. THE WARNING OF THE VIRUS ABOUT US 321

APPENDICES 325

THE COVID-WHIRLPOOL DRAWING 326

LONELY POEM 330

A TALE OF TWO LETTERS ABOUT REMDESIVIR 333

WHY AND HOW TO WEAR A FACE MASK 338

MASKED POETRY 342

FACE MASK MEDITATION 344

MINDING COVID: A DIFFERENT STORY 347

THE FUTURE OF THE COVID STORY 358

NEW STRAIN OR BREXIT STRESS? 360

SIMPLY COVID 362

AN APP TO SUPPORT 364

WHY THE AURELIS APP "CANNOT WORK AGAINST COVID" 366

AFTERWORD 368

ABOUT THE AUTHOR 371

Introduction

This book has been written from March 2020 onwards. The chapters are annotated with the date of my publishing them as blog posts. Each chapter is one post.

The story is not finished. There will be an Edition X of the book in 2021. Hopefully, with good news. Or better: not all too terrible news in view of ongoing pockets of infection or a pending second wave in Europe and the US autumn-winter 2020. Some other parts of the world fare worse.

Much depends on how profoundly the minding-corona premise will be broadly accepted. Apart from what any specific cure (medication, vaccination) may bring, this is about many severely ill patients (with complications over the following years in body and mind) and deaths through not seriously taking the mind into account. On top of this, each corona death is not just any death. So, at the time of writing, the present + recent past has been a disaster. Will the future be another one?

With eyes wide shut, we have been wrecked by a whirlpool in which, apart from the virus, the mind plays a crucial role. Are we bound to be wrecked by that same whirlpool a second time, but with less to no economic reserves to at least save the boat?

I will be angry if that happens. Anger starts with motivational energy. It is with this energy that I am writing this book. The same energy brought about an app that is free for everyone to use that may help in many corona-related situations as well as many other situations of acute stress that leads to symptoms. You can download this free app (android) from https://aurelis.org/aurelis-app and open it on your smartphone. It's also on Google Play and Apple Store.

One might ask why we don't see the mind at work every year during the influenza-season. On the other hand, we may indeed see it at work while not *as working*. Thus, in principle, the ideas of this book may also be applicable to influenza, be it to a lesser degree, at society-level, because we have gotten 'used' to it. Of course, the same applies to the whole domain of psychosomatics (still preferable term). Especially in the subconceptual field, it is difficult to operationalize the investigated patterns into conceptual structures. Isn't it logical? For instance, one may talk about 'anxiety' as a concept. Still, the concept will be interpreted differently by different people. The pattern itself that we talk about as 'anxiety' is even fuzzier.

So, investigating 'anxiety,' we are prone to put quite disparate things in the same box, then examine the influence of the content of this box. For example, if one puts many colors in a box, one gets grey. After having done so, how to investigate the influence of red? The problem is: Reality doesn't stop at such greyish conceptualization. Therefore, we need to make correct distinctions even at the individual level. In the domain of psychosomatics, we are still far from that. This makes it all the more surprising – as we will see in this book – that even while using greyish constructs, we see profound influences of mind on body.

Things are continuously unfolding. The news of yesterday (literally) brought dexamethasone, a long-existing corticosteroid, in the picture as a life-saving drug for many COVID-patients. This may be the best medical news from the medical side until now. Dexamethasone acts through diminishing the immune response. This brings openly, for everyone to see, the importance of the immune system in COVID progression. Is the immune system as important as the virus? Clearly, yes. Is the mind very much intermingled with the immune system? Clearly, yes. Dexamethasone also shows that sometimes a solution to a huge problem may be present nearby and yet hard to notice – until it is noticed. After that, it may change the game and save many lives.

In individuals as well as at society-level, COVID evolves in strange ways that also baffle virologists. Probably it is not the virus that 'acts strangely,' but the host in body-mind unity. Here, we are in a domain in which I am quite knowledgeable. I dare say: more knowledgeable than virologists and most other medical colleagues.

This book is compatible with all available science as far as I can see. We need science. This book adds scientifically to present-day science. In this sense, I dare say that in present-day medical science, we are missing an essential part of ourselves. I have been working on this for the last 20 years. If interested, please see my other books or go to www.aurelis.org. You find a lot of ideas on the blog. Also, in the book, I sometimes directly refer to some blog text. Se:: https://aurelis.org/blog.

If you're not convinced of the power of the mind in matters of health, I invite you to read *Your Mind as Cure*. There, you find a host of theoretical and experimental science backing up this claim, as well as how to put it hands-on into practice for your personal health.

[Note that in writing, to me, unless specifically stated, the masculine is a generic gender.]

Minding Corona – 12 Points

> **The basic 'Minding corona' premise:**
>
> In COVID-19 – the disease progression – the mind is significantly important in cause as well as proper management.
>
> **Probably as important as the virus itself.**

This text is, in 12 points, a 'summary and implications' chapter. In other chapters, I have built an argumentation about the importance of the mind in a multi-causal view of COVID.

About 'mind being important,' I see 'mind' in the broadest sense. Of course, if there is no virus, there is no viral problem. This is black or white. But if the virus is there, in that situation, if you would take out 'mind' from the equation, how would the body react? If you then put 'mind' back into it, but in an optimal way, how would the complete person react? We will never be fully able to do this experiment. It's something to wrap your mind around.

Anyway, seeing 'the virus' as the sole and single cause of what is happening around and more and more also inside many people is clearly wrong. There is always a conglomerate of causes. 'Minding corona' puts significant weight on the mind. This shows that we should concretely take it into account. The implication is huge, although we hardly come across the idea in media. So, from what degree of certainty about the 'Minding corona' premise should we care? In my view:

- From 10% certainty onwards, it is worth putting enough resources into this (worldwide). Compare a few millions of US dollars to billions, trillions.

- From 90% onwards and with properly and practically taking the mind into account, the social cure (economic shutdown, people in lock-down) may be worse than the disease. This is: it lessens the need for a shutdown. What to do, becomes a political decision.

- I'm at 80% and mounting.

Here are the 12 points (of course, in many ways incomplete for the sake of conciseness):

1. The virus is real. The infection is real. The human immune system is real. A substan tial influence of the mind over the immune system is real. Also real is that we do not know how many 'corona deaths' would have occurred without the virus at all. Until further notice, let's agree this is negligible.

2. Body and mind are not two separate entities. Instead, they are two ways of looking at the same thing (human being). "Can the mind influence the body?" is not even a proper question. Of course!

3. The *nocebo phenomenon* is real. This is: the mind can have a negative influence on the body. Given strong expectations and suggestive messages, this influence can be substantial.

4. The 'fight against the virus' continues inside each infected person, related to his immune system, influenced by the mind.

5. Because of the mass psychological happening, it is also a global issue, a 'global hysteria.' The global character heightens the suggestive power.

6. Several elements together enter into a whirlpool in which a person can get very ill and even drown. Panic/hysteria is a

substantial part of this whirlpool. Subconceptual processing (see my book Your Mind as Cure) is intrinsic to this. Towards and within the whirlpool, together with other elements, nocebo can be deadly.

7. With proper means, the help we can give to any individual patient can go far. To many, this may be a question of life or death.

8. We have no precise idea about the death toll of the COVID-virus on its own, in 'normal' no-stress circumstances. We should be – ethically – prepared for any eventuality. The future may show that we are overlooking mind to an inhumane degree at present. Of course, in view of what you are reading, this is to me especially important.

9. The only way to approach 100% certainty is through lots of formalized real-world evidence and the use of A.I. to gather and manage this. Such will be possible in the near future.

10. Panic is never a good advisor. It may be dangerous by itself in two ways at present: 1) collateral damage via economy and lockdown stress (depression, aggression, abandonment), and 2) pushing ill and vulnerable patients over a potentially deadly tipping point.

11. Media communications are also influential. They should neither lead to carelessness nor panic. Images of doom may not be appropriate.

12. Support has been developed as an app that can help people in situations of acute stress, whether caregivers, caretakers or anyone else. This includes people diagnosed with COVID. An even more in-depth answer can be the A.I. driven tool 'Lisa' [see: "Lisa"], diagnostically and therapeutically. Lisa can alleviate through coaching, diminishing panic and heightening motivation. Lisa may also be used in many other domains in the future. This can save economy and many lives.

Note that in case of a correct 'Minding corona' premise, if not taken into account, the danger is no less than at present, irrespective of the final number of deaths. The whirlpool doesn't miraculously disappear. However, the way to handle it is very different. On top of 'the fight against the virus,' we should delve into how we can boost a person's inner defenses *mentally*. More future-oriented, we should delve into who we are, where we stand, where we are heading as a human species. This stressful time is also a proper time to start doing this on a global scale.

1. Pandemia or Global Hysteria?

March 18, 2020

	Today	Total
Cases worldwide	20.736	218.985
Deaths worldwide	983	8.983

This chapter is dedicated to Dr. Li, not because he stood up to Chinese authority but because he stood up. There is hope for humanity as long as there are individuals who are brave enough to stand up, be it in America, in Europe, in Russia, in China or anywhere else.

WARNING: If the psyche is not properly taken into account in this epidemic, we run the risk that this negligence will demand much surplus health-related suffering, many bankruptcies, and a large death toll in the near future. Action should be taken by studying this as a serious possibility.

At the moment, the world has turned corona.

Everybody knows 'the virus.' COVID-19 stands for **CO**rona-**VI**rus **D**isease, 20**19**. This tiniest organism gives a beating to the masters of the universe; namely, us.

It started in Wuhan. It is taking the world. Many people are dying. Western economy may go down the drain in one, two or several waves. The future will be post-corona. Generations from now, people will associate this time with this virus. Nevertheless, might the issue, including its physical effect (influence mind-body), be substantially infested by – with all due respect – 'mass hysteria'?

This is mainly about the evolution from infection to disease. Since it is global by now, it may be the first case of such global hysteria. I do not claim that this is absolutely certain. But well enough, as absurd as it may seem. Likewise, the earth is not flat, and it's not the center of the universe, although both were once preposterous hypotheses.

Causality is tricky to pinpoint. It's like water leaking through your roof and you don't know where the leak is. It may be something you didn't expect, not what you took for granted at first sight. Might the 2020 Corona pandemic be a giant leak through humanity's rooftop at an unexpected place?

Meanwhile, we should continue on the track of extreme caution. Very much is at stake: many people's lives and livelihoods. Therefore, we should investigate every possibility. This is no time for cowardice. This article is not a discussion for being right or wrong. It is a plea for not leaving any possibility blank.

Hysteria?

Global hysteria is not a strictly negative term. There is no reason to this, unless you see anything related to 'non-conscious mental processing' as basically negative. But of course, hysteria is not fear (cause being rather conscious). It's anxiety (final cause being non-conscious). It is not rational. It's irrational. The panic that we see now may come from our living above an underground sea of anxiety. It is a broader lesson we should take from this happening, since it will return in many ways if left unmanaged.

This has a further consequence: people are not guilty for getting the disease after being infected, even while the mind would appear to be deeply involved. Talking about 'guilt' may hinder one's taking responsibility. 'Guilt' should be avoided at all cost! And rationally seen, that is also correct. Moreover, the feeling of responsibility may slow down the progression from infection to disease as it does in others.

This would not be the first example of mass hysteria with an adverse effect on health. Such an outcome is called a 'nocebo.' The mechanism is comparable to that of a true placebo: thoughts influence health and healing, possibly to a huge extent. We see amazing things in the world of placebo, including more and more even in surgery and with objective outcomes. Nowadays, placebogenic effects are being visualized within the brain. Intriguingly, when a person believes in some cure, we see a degree of placebo. When his physician also believes in it, we see more placebo. When the whole environment believes in it, the effect is highest. What if the entire world gets into a craze?

Cases of mass hysteria with consequences on health have been reported from the Middle Ages onward and well into recent years. For instance, in October 2019, at Starehe Girls Centre, Kenya, 68 students were isolated, showing symptoms of cough, sneezing, and low-grade fever, later concluded to be a case of mass hysteria. Another example is the Emirates Flight 203 case in September 2018, in which 106 of 521 passengers on a 14-hour flight from Dubai to New York reported symptoms of coughing, sneezing, fever, or vomiting. The plane was quarantined in New York; only a few passengers turned out to have a common cold.

Common sense?

During 1400 years, in the Western world, the whole of authoritative medicine strongly believed in Galenic theories: four humors, blood suckers, venipunctures, scarifications and weirder stuff, until +/- AD 1800. Fortunately, we live in more scientific times but still far from the optimum. So, imagine going back 300 years and trying to convince the medical world that they are wrong *in total* within some subdomain. Good luck... Of course, this imaginative exercise proves nothing. It lets you feel something. Follow common sense, not necessarily common assumptions.

Mathematical models show a predictable curve of COVID cases within several countries. Does this contradict the premise? I don't think so. Of course, there is infection. No doubt about that. A virus is a virus. The number of infections by this virus is not the core of the 'Minding corona' premise. There is no contradiction. Crucial is why and how many of these infections lead to illness and up to fatality. Moreover, in cases of (post)traumatic stress – somehow also being a kind of hysteria – over an entire population, one can see a curve that waxes and wanes much like the models of the coronavirus show. An example is the number of heart attacks related to the scud rocket strikes by Iraq on Israel in 1991. As always, due to exceptions, any models of this kind should be taken with ample reservation.

Hysteria can spread. Can it spread globally? Possibly, mobiles and mobility play a role. Social media can hype anything and to a huge degree. Air travel brings many people closer to each other, also heightening the idea of global vulnerability.

To many people, it may seem absurd that the mind would have such a profound influence on the body. The idea of 'Mind-Body Divide' still plays a huge role in the acceptance of such. Well, scientifically, we are way beyond that. Absurdity has given way to reality. There is no such divide.

Also, the mind can kill.

You don't need voodoo for that. For instance, we know scientifically that psychosocial stress has a substantial effect on cardiovascular disease (Interheart study, 30.000 subjects, published in the Lancet 2004, showing a ratio of 2.67 increase) and definitely may lead to a heightened grade of premature cardiovascular deaths. We also definitely know that the mind can influence the immune system. There is no doubt. We should have much respect for our minds! After all, isn't that great?

So, can it kill? Yes, and even more if you look at it this way: Within a population, there are always gradations of vulnerability, shades of gray instead of black and white. This includes pneumological and immunological vulnerability. If something lifts the whole curve just a bit higher towards serious disease and fatality, then we see additional cases. Note that raising the curve a little for many people is all that is needed. Can global hysteria do that? This begs for mathematical confirmation.

Of course, people don't 'just die from hysteria.' They may die from a compound of factors in which the mind plays some role. Even with a little role but over a large part of the population, statistical numbers may be substantial. Likewise, while the media talk about 'corona deaths,' people don't just die from corona but from a compound of factors. Within this complex compound, what is the role of corona and what is the role of mind? These are the questions of this article. In any case, I see no proof that corona plays the bigger role. A small sentence. A gigantic consequence.

In many cases in which corona-infected people die from pneumonia complications, the prime killer is not the virus but the immune reaction against it. This causes what is called a 'cytokine storm.' Cytokines are small molecules that are part of the immune response. The storm may damage lung tissue, produce coughing and even lead to pneumonia. Little children do not yet produce many cytokines, which is probably why they usually don't get very sick from the virus.

Scientifically, we know enough about the influence of the mind on immune functions to see a correlation up to mortality. For instance, from HIV-infection to AIDS disease, it is scientifically known – repeatedly proven – that the psyche plays a substantial role. Very likely, it also plays a role in the COVID-case (from real infection to real symptoms and fatality). We have no idea of how significant this role may be.

The panic is a certainty. The media are sowing dire news every minute of the day. Social media are pushing the alarm through the rooftop. 'The virus' is the enemy, the unknown killer. The symptoms of a low-grade COVID-infection are very unspecific. Almost everyone has such symptoms at least once a year. So, everybody is attentive to oneself and others. The incubation period of up to 13 days adds to the unknown. Shops are closed. Bars are closed. Elite scientists are convinced. Everybody is convinced.

The path to global hysteria

How, then, could global hysteria have started? One guess. Wuhan is a highly air-polluted region with many people's airways already damaged, thus vulnerable to viruses and more. With the fear of 'new SARS, only much more infectious' also being a topic in medical circles, the stage was set. Note that in other cases of mass hysteria, the origin can be pinpointed to one or a few people. It needs the right circumstances.

The fatality rate has been much higher in Wuhan than in the rest of China. One reason may be that this is precisely the reason why this mass hysteria has become a global hysteria. This is: because the energy was so high in Wuhan, it could spread so violently. Most unfortunately, the 34-year-old Dr. Li, who blew the whistle but was subdued at first, tragically 'died from corona.' His death was highly mediatized.

Soon, the media took it to heart, showing people being treated by something like spacemen. The most dramatic pictures are the most successful ones: a poor older woman surrounded by several spacemen. Very impressive! Different media feel that, after all, the scarier the news, the more they sell. It's a mechanism. Also, how does the woman feel by this? I would be 'scared to death' by such setting in her place. In any case, it's a perfect environment for high nocebo.

If indeed hysteria is involved, then the global character is utterly amazing. At the same time, it is this global character that may, at present, be fueling the hysteria. We are all subject to draconian measures. It is continuously in the news. The economy might go down. Soon, most people might be in social isolation. It is a perfect environment for global hysteria.

Most important may be to know not who gets the disease, but who doesn't. Due to limited testing material, people at risk (symptoms, contacts, vulnerability) are tested exclusively. A number of them test positive and are treated as COVID-19 diseased. How many of these are infected and have symptoms but with no relation between infection and symptoms? We don't know.

The disease spreads very quickly. This may be caused by modern human mobility. It may also be because the virus is already globally present more than expected, as are its siblings. The future will tell, when we can examine many people's saliva and tissues from before the virus had reached their very specific habitat. The present testing – by way of genetic sequencing – is performed mostly on symptomatic people. Many tests are negative. Some are said to be false negative, which is normal. Unfortunately, we cannot test everyone for the presence of the virus. Many people may be infected unknowingly.

Let's hope there will soon be an antibody test. If this shows many people to be immune already, it may attenuate the panic. At present, there is no such test. We advise putting huge resources into developing one.

Why is there still little spread of the disease in Africa, even in spite of much air traffic from China? Natural immunity? Lack of testing? Young population? Less of this hysteria? With measles and malaria, there is indeed less reason to see the new virus as the most dreadful enemy. It's 'just' one of several deadly infections. This might say more about the rest of the world than about Africa itself. Africa saw a relatively large death burden from the 2009 H1N1 Influenza (not Corona) pandemic. There was no specific invulnerability back then; quite the contrary. The difference may be one between somatic and psychological causal factors. The 2009 Influenza pandemic had an overall estimated global fatality of 152.000 – 575.000, mostly in low-income countries. We are still far from that, but the panic is much bigger, mainly in high-income countries.

In China, meanwhile, the epidemic power is already declining. This is scientifically noteworthy. Have many people become immune to the virus? Or to the hysteria? Probably both?

Several strains of coronavirus exist. Some are dangerous; most are benign. SARS, MERS... many people have been psychologically sensitized by stories of viruses (including Ebola) with a much higher fatality rate. One should indeed be watchful for a pandemic of a kind of synthesis of Ebola and the common cold. I mean: a virus with an unfortunate combination of characteristics of both. In that case, the disaster is unimaginable. The possibility exists. We should be prepared! The unknown makes the case of COVID-19 scarier. It appears to be of the more dangerous kind, but not as dangerous as SARS or MERS in the percentage of fatality among the infected.

Yet panic is never a good advisor.

Sowing panic for political gain is ethically wrong. We also see that not many influential people dare to row against the current. This is understandable, but it creates a hyperbole of additional panic. Nobody wants to be the guy who was less cautious than the other guy. OK, but imposing panic is not readily the preferable way to make people more cautious. For one thing, if the acute panic has gone, so has the motivation to remain cautious. This may be essential in forming a second wave. If panic is then again crucial to make people cautious, it will also again fuel the next whirlpool.

Streams of information about fatality rates may cause part of the hysteria. Well, people die. Strangely, we have become less used to living with death. Strangely, the media talk about fatality rates as if death is something uncommon. It is not. Not even your smartphone makes you invulnerable.

One might object that this pandemic comes after the Influenza season, in which normally seen, weaker persons may have already died. So, this pandemic seems worse. I agree with this only partly. People may be weakened by Influenza, now getting a second hit. I remember working in a Brazilian favela where uncomplicated measles had a high fatality rate among undernourished children. Moreover, in the case of hysteria, there is a vulnerability of a different kind. If next winter, corona comes on top of influenza, the disaster may be even bigger.

Part of the present *obvious* hysteria shows in how people storm to shops to buy lots of stuff they may personally need without any thought of the common good. In any case, this doesn't show the best side of the human being. Natural disasters generally unite people; pandemics may sometimes rather divide people. Why is this so? Are people egoistic in the first place, then also a bit altruistic 'for the good feeling of it'? Perhaps. In my view, this is what makes us prone to global hysteria, be it this one or the next.

Yes, I am quite sure there will be a future global hysteria of the kind. The world is getting smaller. 'Global' seems next door. Billions of people provide billions of self-broadcast opinions and, thus, lots of energy for a hysterical global tsunami. Can we learn from this one? This one is about dying. What if the next one is about violent behavior fueled by scarcity, distrust, short-range empathy and disruptions by climate change?

Nothing should be taken for granted.

As proof in the pudding, or at least a step in that direction, I propose the use of an Implicit Association Test (IAT), such as what is available online from Harvard: https://implicit.harvard.edu/implicit/takeatest.html. The COVID-IAT (to be developed) could gauge implicit assumptions about the personal risk to get severely ill or even die from the virus. We can differentiate groups and discern the impact of non-conscious convictions in this matter. This may give a good indication for further investigations.

At present, most people think in one direction, and this is not the direction towards inside. One can see this precisely as an essential part of things unfolding now. Inner dissociation ('not being connected to inside') makes one vulnerable: to manipulative politicians, to burnout, to chronic pain, to addictions; you name it. We have increasingly seen a fair share of this the last few years. Meanwhile, it is indeed very challenging to think out of this box. Everybody – globally! – thinks in one direction, so it is just weird to take another direction. Yet we may have to, not only concerning this crisis but much broader. As said, many problems have been mounting, and they will continue doing so. Maybe the present crisis can be a turning point in getting a grip on this other more existential crisis.

After the acute phase(s), we will see an aftermath that may take many years, well into a generation. Of course, there will be economic aftermath. Also, there will be an aftermath of post-traumatic stress. This can have a huge effect culturally, which from now on, can best be seen as global-culturally. This stress is 'energy:' it leads to change. There will be a lot of it, with huge danger, and a huge possibility to use it constructively. What will it be?

Most of all, let us try to remain rational. We end as we started: concerning COVID, this is as yet a hypothesis; nothing more, nothing less. We should continue being at least as cautious as we are. At the same time, let's research this possibility: In COVID-19 – the disease progression, not the infection – the mind may be more important than the virus in cause as well as proper management.

Some practical to-dos:

- Follow all hygienic advice from a trusted source.

- Get a clear picture of the width of the ideas in this article. Your conscious insight by itself is more valuable than you might think. The non-conscious acts in non-conscious ways. For every person, making an effort towards the best possible insight is invaluable.

- Appreciate the power of your mind as much as possible, even in ways that you are not fully aware of. Stop your activities once in a while and contemplate.

- Contemplate about your mind and body being one. Don't let there be any remaining doubt about this.

- Make a clear distinction between 'infection rate' and 'confirmed infection rate' in your appreciation of morbidity and mortality rates.

- Listen to the news with a critical mind, taking into account what you have just read. Analyze the news for its intent to sell by sowing panic, and talk about this with your family and friends.

- If you are an anchorman, please don't sow panic. There are many ways to bring the news objectively.

- Promote research using IAT as denoted in the article. Play a while with the Harvard test. It's fun and lets you know yourself a bit better. For millennia already, self-knowledge has been seen as the basis of all wisdom. Count inner strength to the latter.

- Each time you wash your hands (many times), also imagine washing your mind. 'The virus' is metaphorically important as well as physically.

- Appreciate your life. Appreciate every day. A trying period may help more than ever.

- Help someone. Do it as if it's the same as helping yourself. In that case, it is.

- And, well, read my book *Your Mind as Cure*.

2. Mind and Corona

March 20, 2020

	Today	Total
Cases worldwide	30.719	275.893
Deaths worldwide	1.380	11.457

Disclaimer: This article is not a scientific review.

Most unfortunately, the disclaimer holds truth.

This article is not a scientific review because there is no science to review.

Optimistically, I went for a search on PubMed 18 March 2020. Searching for 'COVID' and 'coronavirus' separately, the results were as follows:

Search term	Number of articles found
COVID/coronavirus psychosocial	0
COVID/coronavirus depression	0
COVID/coronavirus social stress	0
COVID/coronavirus psychological	0
COVID/coronavirus psychology	0
COVID/coronavirus mental	0

And more desperately:

COVID/coronavirus placebo	0
COVID/coronavirus nocebo	0

[Note that 'coronavirus' also comprises SARS and MERS, separate from COVID-19.]

Also, nothing related that I could think of. The zeros are additionally worrisome because the new coronavirus outbreak causes immense stress on the population worldwide. Panic plays a role in what causes more panic. First, another disclaimer.

Second disclaimer: Nothing in this article carries even the slightest form of disrespect.

This is my second article about mind and corona. People who don't see the role of the mind in the enfolding story may think that 'hard' facts are being denigrated in this. To me, it is the opposite. The hardest fact about the mind is that so little is scientifically known about its influence upon health and healing. Yet even with this little knowledge, already the influence that we see is substantial. We may be blind for an avalanche that is going on and will become visible in due time. In many domains of healthcare, many hard facts together are pointing to this. It is not only possible. It is quite probable.

Anyway, being intrigued by the above zeros, I read a substantial number of scientific articles about many aspects of COVID. In these too, there was no mention of the mind within an ocean of information on physical elements. Even I feel lured by this into a vicious circle: the whole domain doesn't look mind-related because no one mentions it. Therefore, no one mentions it.

One gets the impression of being drawn into a comfortable illusion, a silo devoid of mind. But of course, we know that viral infections (from infestation to disease) are immune-related, and that the immune system is mind-related. There is no doubt about either one. Research is more than clear. This includes — crucial to the present case of COVID — unmistakable proof of influence of acute psychosocial stress on immuno-inflammatory mechanisms in general and as measured in saliva and in the blood. Individuals vary markedly in the magnitude of change, logically, also in relation to age (called 'inflammaging'). Little has been done with this knowledge until now.

So, we don't know, but...

Meanwhile, we are still at the beginning of being able to pinpoint the most relevant aspects. A lot lies in store. Not only the immune system in a strict sense is involved. In humans, acute viral infections often lead to inflammation in the lungs. More and more, stress is also being related to inflammation. Arguably, in extraordinary circumstances, both together may lead to a whirlpool of inflammation and the 'acute respiratory distress syndrome' that is so deadly in COVID-pneumonia.

Another especially stark example of negative clinical outcome is Takotsubo. This is an acute major-stress induced heart disease – also known as broken heart syndrome – with a prognosis comparable to myocardial infarction. The mechanism involves an acute inflammation of the heart muscle. On the other hand, we know that the maintenance of a positive outlook during acute stress protects against pro-inflammatory reactivity. With this in mind, we can have a different look at COVID fatalities. Interesting, in the latter, we also see an unexpected inflammation of the heart muscle in more and more cases.

One expert in personal communication: "If you ask ten virologists, you get ten different opinions about what to do." This is OK; it is science at its best. But it shows what it is. Science, especially about people, seldom gives one definite answer. For politicians, this is a puzzle. They follow the experts' advice, but which ones of the experts? One needs to take into account what seems absurd at first sight. I do have great admiration for virologists. They know much about coronaviruses. But about the human mind? Of course, 'no knowledge' doesn't mean there is nothing present. It's like with eyes closed, saying there is nothing to see. It's not comfortable.

Coming up with the psyche is even dangerous – career-wise – in a somato-scientific milieu. What about now? "This is not the time to come forward with such. People have serious things to attend to." Of course, this is *precisely* the time to take every possible measure. It is never more necessary. Also, a crisis may set things in motion that would otherwise not occur.

Therefore, let's talk about the mind.

At least, we know something about the influence of the mind on viral infections and disease. Since the nineties, AIDS research of high scientific level has shown a substantial impact of the mind on the progression from virus-infestation to AIDS. I describe this in my book *Your Mind as Cure*, together with research by Cohen about the influence of psychic stress on the incidence of common colds after viral contact, even in a direct dose-response relationship. Note that among the common cold viruses, several are of the corona type, although, of course, much less dangerous than the COVID-19 virus. I also describe a lot of scientifically proven influences of the mind on many symptoms and diseases, including immune-related ones. In fact, medical research is brimming with all this if one cares to look for it.

I want to share a few quotes, not as causal proof but as a strong wake-up:

- "The studies summarized in this review indicate that there are important linkages between anxiety and depression and viral diseases such as influenza A (H1N1) and other influenza viruses, varicella-zoster virus, herpes simplex virus, human immunodeficiency virus/acquired immune deficiency syndrome, and hepatitis C." [Coughlin SS. Anxiety and Depression: Linkages with Viral Diseases. *Public Health Rev.* 2012;34(2):92.]

- "In the Swedish population, stress related disorders were associated with a subsequent risk of life threatening infections, after controlling for familial background and physical or psychiatric comorbidities." [Song H, Fall K, Fang F, et al. Stress related disorders and subsequent risk of life threatening infections: population based sibling controlled cohort study. *BMJ.* 2019;367:l5784.]

- "These data demonstrate support for the effectiveness of stress-reducing psychological interventions in improving immunity in studies that tested immune function by means of incorporating an in vivo, in vitro, or psychophysiological challenge." [Schakel L, Veldhuijzen DS, Crompvoets PI, et al. Effectiveness of Stress-Reducing Interventions on the Response to Challenges to the Immune System: A Meta-Analytic Review. *Psychother Psychosom*. 2019;88(5):274–286.]

- "Social disruption (SDR) is a well-characterized mouse stressor that causes changes in immune cell reactivity in response to inflammatory stimuli. In this study, we found that SDR in the absence of an immune challenge induced pulmonary inflammation." [Curry JM, Hanke ML, Piper MG, et al. Social disruption induces lung inflammation. Brain Behav Immun. 2010;24(3):394–402.]

- "The present report meta-analyzes more than 300 empirical articles describing a relationship between psychological stress and parameters of the immune system in human participants. Acute stressors (lasting minutes) were associated with potentially adaptive upregulation of some parameters of natural immunity and downregulation of some functions of specific immunity. Brief naturalistic stressors (such as exams) tended to suppress cellular immunity while preserving humoral immunity. Chronic stressors were associated with suppression of both cellular and humoral measures." [Segerstrom SC, Miller GE. Psychological stress and the human immune system: a meta-analytic study of 30 years of inquiry. Psychol Bull. 2004;130(4):601–630.]

- "Cortisol also showed a continuous association with duration of viral shedding, an indicator of viral replication and continuing infection, such that higher cortisol concentrations predicted more days of shedding." [Janicki-Deverts D, Cohen S, Turner RB, Doyle WJ. Basal salivary cortisol secretion and susceptibility to upper respiratory infection. *Brain Behav Immun*. 2016;53:255–261.]

- "Both aging processes and psychological stress affect the immune system: Each can dysregulate immune function with a potentially substantial impact on physical health. Worse, the effects of stress and age are interactive." [Graham JE, Christian LM, Kiecolt-Glaser JK. Stress, age, and immune function: toward a lifespan approach. *J Behav Med.* 2006;29(4):389–400. doi:10.1007/s10865-006-9057-4]

- "Stress-induced immune dysregulation has been shown to be significant enough to result in health consequences, including reducing the immune response to vaccines, slowing wound healing, reactivating latent herpesviruses, such as Epstein-Barr virus (EBV), and enhancing the risk for more severe infectious disease." [Godbout JP, Glaser R. Stress-induced immune dysregulation: implications for wound healing, infectious disease and cancer. *J Neuroimmune Pharmacol.* 2006;1(4):421–427.]

- "This study supports the hypothesis that maternal psychological stress affects the inflammatory response in their allergic children." [Tsuji M, Koriyama C, Yamamoto M, Anan A, Shibata E, Kawamoto T. The association between maternal psychological stress and inflammatory cytokines in allergic young children. *PeerJ.* 2016;4:e1585.]

- "Importantly, we concluded that nocebo studies outline how individual expectations may lead to physiological changes underpinning the central integration and processing of magnified pain signaling. Further research is needed to develop strategies." [Blasini M, Corsi N, Klinger R, Colloca L. Nocebo and pain: An overview of the psychoneurobiological mechanisms. *Pain Rep.* 2017;2(2):e585.]

- "Stress is an external factor known to be a potent exacerbator of respiratory infections. Most explanations of how stress affects susceptibility to airway infections focus on the immune system. However, evidence is increasing that respiratory pathogens are equally responsive to the hormonal output of stress." [Stover

CM. Mechanisms of Stress-Mediated Modulation of Upper and Lower Respiratory Tract Infections. *Adv Exp Med Biol.* 2016;874:215–223.

- "Media reports about the adverse effects of supposedly hazardous substances can increase the likelihood of experiencing symptoms following sham exposure and developing an apparent sensitivity to it." [Witthöft M, Rubin GJ. Are media warnings about the adverse health effects of modern life self-fulfilling? An experimental study on idiopathic environmental intolerance attributed to electromagnetic fields (IEI-EMF). *J Psychosom Res.* 2013;74(3):206–212.]

And on and on... Psychoneuroimmunology thrives.

Focusing on the COVID issue, I see people being careless in what they call 'infected persons.' In most cases, they mean 'positively tested persons.' Following this scheme of those who get infected:

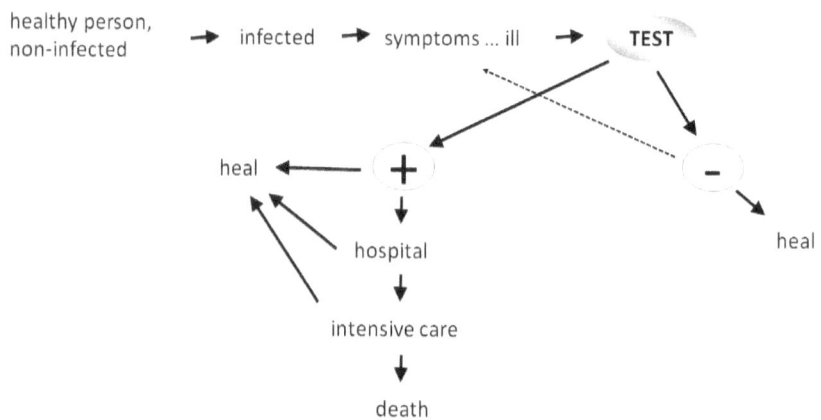

Note that the test is not a test of COVID-disease – of course – but of infestation. People get ill from a compound of causes, to which the test is not necessarily related in a straightforwardly causal way:

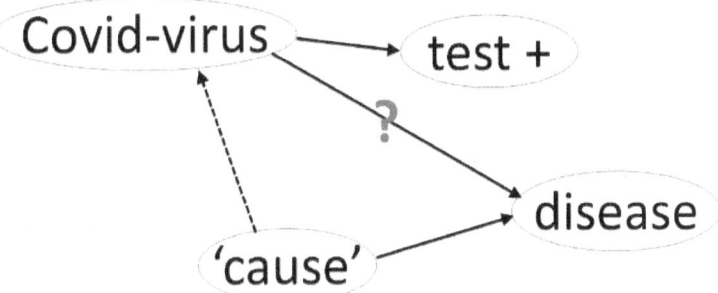

What might be the mysterious 'cause'?

Now for a bold assumption...

Perhaps most importantly, the question is: Can someone, through massive suggestion (the 'global hysteria' from my first article) become heavily immune-labile in the short term? In two directions:

- On the one hand, that of a shutdown (immunosuppression)
- On the other hand, a 'storm' such as we see now in the case of COVID-19: a 'cytokine storm' that in chaos is not necessarily focused on one pathogen or an element of the own tissue, but rather flies to all directions at the same time. Compare it with general anxiety syndrome.

Or both: first the one, then the other?

Theoretically, yes. Science speaks in COVID-cases of an immune response out of control. And if it can be the case for one or a few, it can be the case for many. Of course, the virus is there, but that is not yet proof that it plays the central role. The primary role may be psychological. In principle, the virus might be no more than a gateway.

How dare I utter such an idea in this time of horror? Rationally speaking, precisely because of the latter. The horror is immense for those directly involved. That *may* have a devastating result on the immune systems of many. I am aware of the hardness of this message at present in a domain with few certainties. Tears fill my eyes while writing. But what if it's true? As hard as I try, I cannot disprove it.

The present panic is a very suggestive one, focused on the lungs and terrible pictures and a horrible death – to many also a 'lonely death.' One shouldn't see this as the power of panic, but of some kind of in-depth chaos, of which the panic is part. It's not that a person freaks out and then even more and then goes through the roof inside, and that's it. Reality is much more open-complex and multidimensional. Looking at the panic just as such is looking past the meaningfulness of human being.

Note that the illness starts with unspecific symptoms: a bit of fever, sore throat, coughing. Attention is drawn to the cough and the fear of 'having the virus.' Then the coughing becomes more and more pronounced, putting a strain on bronchi and lungs. Through this and several stress-related pathways – which have scientifically been investigated – they get inflamed. It becomes worse. 'Ground-glass pneumonia' may become visible on radiography of the lungs (but not necessarily even in a fully symptomatic patient).

The person is put in quarantine. Rightly so, but it immensely heightens the stress levels of all concerned: themselves, health workers, loved ones, the general public. The ill person may get more and more caught in a hugely meaning-replete pattern of pending doom. Compare it to a whirlpool in which one can get caught and drown. The mental influence may not seem like much from a distance, but when you get inside...

The person gets tested at some stage, and COVID-virus is found. That can surely not be 'psychogenic'... Indeed. Virus is virus. But look at the test: some patients with severe symptoms had to be tested six times before the virus was found. According to scientific literature, there have to be symptoms before the test can be positive. Some people are false-positive, then negative, then positive. It seems there are many holes in this testing at present. Even so, of course, viruses are never 'psychogenic,' but that is beside the point. It helps, though, to keep people – including experts – dramatically away from the point.

At the therapy side, the viruses are not attacked through present-day treatment. People recover from inside, with external support of their life systems. This means that there is no proof through eradication of the virus. In other words, there is as yet no infallible proof that the virus plays the central role.

One may rightfully ask: Can the mind, in principle, be invisible to such a degree? Yes. For instance, arthroscopic operations for osteoarthritis of the knee have been performed in the US on approximately 650.000 patients each year with good results. A double-blind study in 2002 revealed no difference with placebo operations. Thus: the effect of the mind. Point is: This discrepancy was not seen during the years before 2002, not by patients, nor by physicians, in spite of the six digit number of cases. How come?

People believe in science.

But science is not a belief. Many people believe in it as if it were one. So, if 'science' points in a specific direction, then that is sometimes taken for granted in a way that contradicts the basis of science itself, which lies in always remaining critical. Scientists – like everybody else – need to struggle against a propensity to thrive in 'science as a belief.' Especially in a crisis such as the present one, true science lies in staying open to every possibility. We don't need less science. We need more.

If there is a substantial mental factor involved in COVID-19, then *not* taking this adequately into account means that many more (than need be) infected people get sicker and thus also more infectious. Through this, the panic heightens and the vicious circle gets stronger. Many more of the infected people may die. It is absurd *not* to take this into account. Yet, it may be hard for a somatic thinker to get into a psychological mind frame since he is used to *seeing* and *handling* the things of importance — for instance, a virus. The deeper mind – especially in its overlap with the body – is not visible. Culturally, we live in a continuous cognitive illusion, acting as if it's not there. Also, in practice, there is still a lot of unicausal thinking around. With a preference for the body, the mind falls overboard

Jean-Luc Mommaerts

3. The Message in the Virus

March 22, 2020

	Today	Total
Cases worldwide	**32.483**	**337.869**
Deaths worldwide	**1.638**	**14.739**

Involuntary messenger

OK. I've asked myself: Why not wait to bring this message until the worst part of the pandemic is over? It's an inconvenient message. Nevertheless:

- 'Panic' kills. It does so mainly by being an additional risk factor. If spread over large populations, the absolute numbers may become substantial. Panic grows panic, and before you know it, you have a forest of panic, especially if the enemy is worldwide and invisible, a dark killer.

- Panic is always a bad advisor. We should not give in to that, just like that. Draconian measures, yes, with a non-panicky message. Panic makes a society vulnerable. Moreover, it demotivates many — arguably, especially adolescents, by nature. We should be motivating people from their inner strength and make panic unneeded. Fortunately, this is partly happening.

- Now is the best time to investigate the issue in prospective studies. It would be interesting to measure stress levels (blood or saliva) in the whole population. Not feasible now, but we can quickly make it so. One can then perform an ongoing study to look for correlations between stress levels and subsequent illness and mortality. Now is the time to do this, for instance, in Lombardy, Italy. This is not about using people as mere subjects in a study. It's about giving sense to suffering. If we see a clear relationship even after a few days, then already, we can take appropriate action, saving lives.

- Large populations (Africa, India, with inadequate healthcare facilities for many) may still be at the beginning of this pandemic, whatever the factors involved. We should do everything possible to mitigate this.

- If the psyche plays a crucial role, how are we going to mourn the preventable deaths of loved ones if we don't act on it now? How would you ever get over it?

- Shortening the pandemic by one week is already worthwhile in saving lives and in saving economically.

My conclusion is that we should not wait to take this to heart until the first big wave has subsided. That would be utterly inhumane. Things can be done now.

Ongoing story

While writing this series of articles, events are unfolding worldwide. In China, the levels of new cases and mortality rates have plummeted. The drastic measures and social discipline may have prevented a giant disaster. They _may_ mainly have had a psychologically soothing effect, explaining the relatively quick national recovery. With an eye on the mind, now is the time to investigate this. By nature, Chinese people would surely be glad to assist – or take the lead. Please, do!

In the West, the communication is suboptimal. I mainly hear this message: "It will be awful if we don't follow the measures with huge discipline, and many people don't." This is a well-meant message of doom, which should be avoided.

With utmost respect, I dread to mention that the cases of Italy and Iran – and Spain in the following – fit the picture: these are emotional cultures, praise to them! But it may make them more acutely vulnerable to extreme circumstances such as the present one. This may make them the 'first responders' in a negative sense, of things to come elsewhere. There is no proof in this, but an eerie correlation. Reading about Iran: "... thanks to a lack of international aid, government mismanagement, and nobody knowing quite who's in charge." (www.dw.com/en/iran-faces-catastrophic-death-toll-from-coronavirus/a-52811895)

In this, I read 'panic.'

Of course, there are other factors, such as sanctions on Iran, leading to a shortage of medical supplies. In the case of Lombardy, I read they were tossed from odd carelessness to terror and panic. Italians are a very outgoing people. The political message in Italy, right now, is also one of terror (terrorizing) and panic. At the same time, carelessness of individuals is mediatized. Meanwhile, in the public's eye, the 'message from Italy to Europe' is that we all need to be extremely wary and still, disaster will probably sweep over the continent.

Differentiating, at this moment, Germany from Italy+Spain. The vast difference (2 vs. 113 deaths per million inhabitants) also intrigues specialists. The 'whirlpool phenomenon' may play a substantial role. According to this, Italy fell in the rut (whirlpool) head-on and seems not yet to be getting out of it. Germany has stayed out of it. Among other things, from the beginning, a huge amount of testing showed real numbers of disease rates. This information calmed the population and became 'self-fulfilling' by keeping them out of the whirlpool. Put on top of this a firm and non-dramatizing leadership.

It is, of course, difficult to prove/disprove the 'whirlpool phenomenon.' That's why we should investigate it now for future's sake. In the meantime, the relevant future may be very near to some parts of the world. In that case, there is no time to waste. Unfortunately, I see the elements coming together for the UK and the US.

In cities: people need to come out of their houses for food and other supplies, of course. It's more difficult to keep social distance. That's also what city dwellers see happening in many places: people still gathering on streets, in transportation, in parks. That may be additionally scary to many. The "virus is in the air."

Back to Africa. Why is the death rate so much lower in Africa currently and so much higher in the West? Around 2 million Chinese live and work on the African continent. There was no ban on air travel to Africa until well too late. The virus is also there. Are Africans lucky this time, as some experts say, or does the cause of the differential perhaps lie in the West? Meanwhile, in the cases of Africa, India and Latin-America, the situation is hugely dangerous.

Remember the thesis of this book: a whirlpool containing several factors including, prominently, the mind. One particular factor may be inherent to social media. Its A.I.-driven, self-learning algorithms are continuously trying to optimize click-bait. These algorithms 'know' that scary stuff sells more. Also, they 'know' how to influence people towards becoming better customers, say, even more readily anxious. Note that this can be done automatically without any person's evil intent.

This process is well-known. The result is always the same: people are made anxiety-prone. When a storm comes over the world, it's put upon this field of anxiety. Freaking out people heightens click-bait. It also increases massive responses that can result in immune imbalances. A bubble of the-scarier-the-more-successful envelops the planet. On top of this, people generally seem to get more dissociated from their inner being. This leads to increasing levels of burnout, depression, chronic pain, general anxiety, etc. It may also heighten the vulnerability of whole groups to catastrophic reactions in their immune system. Note, in this respect, that the immune system and the central nervous system are closely integrated and are even of the same origin. We 'think' also with our immune system.

Causal elements

I see some further causes of this widespread vulnerability: a shortening of attention span, massive consumption of antidepressants – of which we don't know how they work, but they surely diminish inner communication, lessening of contact with nature, 'rationalization' standing in the way of poetry. Also: losing a deep sense of meaningfulness, losing openness, human respect, and trust, losing the freedom just to be oneself. As I keep repeating: There is no guilt in this. Some people and groups of people are by nature more sensitive (say: humanely warm) and may thereby also be more vulnerable, especially in extraordinary circumstances. It just makes it all the more poignant.

With this in mind, in social media at least, anyone can take care in his small part of the world. In social 3D, one can be friendly at a 'social distance.' Smiling does not infect anyone. On the other hand, friendliness – at all levels, from personal to highest diplomacy – may affect anyone's immune system and level of low-grade inflammation. The viruses are a scientific reality; this also. If we can see it as a step towards a better, more humane future, then even people in acute respiratory distress may look forward to this, which may help them to survive.

Whoever thinks this is nonsense is not a wise – although possibly an intelligent – person. A truly empathic attitude towards all is recommended. For instance, in shops, to the ones who work there. This is no sheer altruism. By being friendly, there is a better chance that you get friendliness in return. That may boost your immune system.

Our minds

The present is a good turning point to better respect our minds for the sake of 'the universe inside' and all the positive this can bring. There is a lot to do. For instance, the concept of 'empathy' is by itself immensely more complex than is generally thought, including in scientific circles! Social media should be studied much more with a critical eye towards this. Right now, we can make people aware. Try to take energy out of the eruption without demotivating anyone to take all possible measures against viral infection! This is a positive-message motivation. We still have a lot to learn. A message of discipline is crucial. Sowing panic may even have the reverse effect on this.

Of course, the enormity of the present problem grabs me too. Is it conceivable that thousands of people have already died and many more will probably die from a 'compound of problems' in which the mind plays a significant role, while almost entirely *not* being adequately taken into account? Is it thus conceivable that the mind plays a more significant role than the virus in what we see happening now? Scientifically, we cannot exclude it. So, we can say with certainty that it is possible. Knowing a substantial part of the research, I would say it's even probable. That is still not a certainty. But if it is the case, then we are tackling the problem wrongly. We should then not do some of the things we do, and we should do some of the things we don't. For starters, in that case, COVID is a misnomer. It's an important one since it puts all emphasis on the virus and doesn't nudge the patient into self-reliance.

Furthermore, it's interesting to look at the acute respiratory distress syndrome as a whirlpool. Once you are in it, it's hard to get out – hard but still feasible, always feasible. But from a distance, or even at the periphery inside, it's <u>relatively</u> easy to heighten your chances not to get swept further into it when you know how to. The 'relatively' is related to deep meaningfulness, as is the whole domain of psychosocial stress. Therefore, in an absolute sense, it may at the same be an immense challenge.

The first part of the challenge lies in appreciating the strength of the whirlpool from even a small distance. This way, it's also hard to comprehend what can be done to avoid people getting sucked into it. For instance, we should avoid anxiety as a deterrent against irresponsible behavior in a 'war against the virus,' etc.

Responsibility

Of course, we desperately need the responsible behavior itself. The focus should be on protection against 'the virus.' Moreover, providing confidence to others that one is doing whatever is possible to prevent further infestation also has a huge soothing effect. It relieves the panic and helps many towards not getting caught in the whirlpool. Despite social distancing, the message of 'being together' is essential in this age. On the other hand, non-believers-in-the-virus are doing a lousy job twice.

"In my view, a substantial part of the current and coming morbidity and mortality – and economic woes – can be blamed to not sufficiently taking into account the deeply human side of human being, the subject of my Ph.D. Looking back, we face an immense ethical problem." This is a quote from an email that I'm sending to more and more people who can make a difference.

Communication to the public should be honest, trustworthy, open, with due respect to our deeply-human nature. If people trust in something (we are protected, special, immune) and then that starts falling, it may fall heavily. Being a realist, anxiety may help to make people (not everyone) more cautious, but it also adds to the whirlpool. I think it is best to be open to this. That starts with proper insight. As I already pointed out, not so much the panic itself, but the meaning level behind/below it is most important. Internal conviction. This is also crucial for health workers who are working in contact with the acutely ill or dying. This may infest them consciously and even more non-consciously, in this way making them more vulnerable.

A possible message could be: "Avoiding panic, staying relaxed may heighten your internal defense against viral disease. IF the virus enters you, it has less chance to make you seriously ill."

Nearing the end of this writing, I need to point out the following. For instance, in China, 71.000 deaths happen in a year due to Influenza flu. The number of deaths due to COVID is stable at this moment at +/- 3300. Looked at it this way, it almost seems little. But if you take out the 71.000, then the death toll of COVID is still a whopping 3300! Globally, the World Health Organization (WHO) estimates that the Influenza flu kills 290,000 to 650,000 people per year, many of these also in economically developed countries. For instance, in the US, 61,000 deaths were linked to the virus in the 2017-2018 season. If COVID-disease and mortality numbers end up in the range of the seasonal flu – which is yet uncertain at present – then, of course, one still comes on top of the other. However, there is a huge discrepancy between the public/political/economic reactions and fall-out, mainly due to, as said, the *uncertainty*. The economic shutdown is and will be a source of suffering on its own: businesses going bankrupt = people going broke, no money for those in need, etc. This is a massive problem in its own right. The victims are the poor, within nations and between nations.

Who are we?

Crucially, in any case, and also future-oriented, we should learn to understand who we are, especially in the 'universe inside.' We should learn more about our inner strength. This may also be important – even more so – towards the flu and many other diseases. The present heart-wrenching wave can pass without this possibility being taken seriously. Then we will not know what may have happened. On top of the vast human suffering, we will have missed an opportunity for the future.

Ah, the future. It suddenly seems further away than usual. I imagine a post-corona world as a kind of awakening out of a bad dream, and hopefully, an era. I know realism, but I like to dream too. From this coronalia era, we may look forward to a world in which people can be happy with less complicated things — for instance, oneself and a few others. One may learn to be more creative. Another one may learn to appreciate small things and to enjoy the beauty around in spite of anything. We may all realize the better world. Musing about what it can be.

To take care of each other, to not take the care for granted.

To look forward to better moments and find joy in them today.

To take some time in order to have some time instead of throwing it out.

To enjoy what some other person enjoys just because.

To be generous. To let others take as long as they don't take you.

To have enough with less.

To give time, not give it away.

To try and try and never give up.

To be inspiring and see where that leads to, with a smile.

To be able to dream a sweet dream.

4. COVID and Attention

March 28, 2020

	Today	Total
Cases worldwide	**66.919**	**665.092**
Deaths worldwide	**3.672**	**31.835**

Multicausality

Unicausal thinking = having unduly exclusive attention for one cause to any issue. Within multiple possible causes, unicausal thinking searches for the cause that explains the consequence. In the animal world, it is frequently a matter of life or death. If you are potential prey and a predator turns up, then you'd better focus your attention on this one predator, even if there is food available or an attractive mating partner. Innumerous times, unicausal thinking has saved one of your ancestors. You wouldn't be around without it. That explains its power in everyday circumstances. It doesn't make unicausal thinking a rational option in an endeavor to be optimally logical.

Unicausal thinking is embedded in Western medical practice and theory as well as in Western conceptual thinking generally. This, to such a degree that it is regarded as inappropriate to propose a multicausal medical model when involving the mind. In practice, we still live in a mind-body divide. In the case of COVID, medical colleagues may see it as dangerous to even mention the possibility of substantial psychological involvement.

Especially in times of stress – the predator, the human enemy, the virus – the thinking naturally becomes more unicausal. Nevertheless, the rational thing to do is to surpass it radically. Reality is never unicausal. In the human case, the psyche – due to many complex ways of realization – is always in many ways involved.

We should give attention to who we really are as mind-body creatures. Now is a good time to jumpstart that. It is the *message in the virus*. This may seem like detracting attention from the fight against the virus. It may seem like now we need to give our full attention to the damned virus. And that is true. Only, 'our full attention' needs to come from who we really are as a total person. It fully should be 'our attention.' This may immediately save lives. If the 'Minding corona' premise is correct, then it is perilous not to take it into account **as soon as possible**. Then it is not so much the '**co**rona **vi**rus **d**isease' (COVID) as it is 'our disease.'

In unicausal thinking, the search for the cure tends to be oriented to one cause. An efficient anti-specific-virus drug would cure COVID. Take the pill and get back to work (family, local bar, tourist destination). I see two main objections: 1) We don't have that pill, and 2) It would again go past the reality of ourselves. It would prolong 'our disease.'

Forming decisions about social measures, scientific experts are consulted. In times of COVID, the sought-after expertise is mainly virus-oriented, at the fringe somewhat psyche-oriented. It should be both without distraction. Within a proper synthesis, they will *both* be more effective.

Of course, we should not lessen the search for the pill, nor the vaccine. Also, we should be prepared for an even worse 'common-cold Ebola' virus to appear sooner or later. Likewise, we should not lessen the search for our deeper self.

Attention

The chapter after this one is about what to do. The main thing in any of that is doing it with attention that you feel coming from deep inside yourself.

Here, of course, lies a difficult distinction between superficial and deep attention. Western culture has become caught in a stream of superficial attention, with 'no time to waste' in production and consumption. Social media have become extremely speedy media. A marketeer should 'grab the prospect' from the first three-two-one seconds, or the prospect is gone. Sadly, handling the prospect this way also makes him this way, especially if many marketers perform the same trick over and over again. With the advent of A.I. in social media, the pace is only accelerating. Hmm. Is my opinion an exaggeration?

Now for the not-so-easy distinction, a primer:

- **superficial attention**: to the symptom, for instance, carrying at first not much more information content than its description in a medical textbook. On top of this can come information and emotionality that is not embedded within yourself. Superficial attention more readily tears you away from your inner strength.

- deep attention: being more open to many associations at the same time. In this way, one can see broader patterns that are not visible when looking at each of them separately. Deep attention is more 'parallel' in contrast to superficial attention being more serial. This brings an openness that lies not so much in what is seen but in the seer. Through the symptom, deep attention is more sensitive to what lies behind or beneath it. Deep attention leads you more readily to your inner strength. If you are a genuinely religious person, you may somewhat recognize this feeling.

Many people can use guidance on how to make the distinction. However, eventually, you can be your own best guide in giving it the best you can and put this into practice, again and again.

Wondering how

Wondering how a 'global hysteria' might become so powerful at present – more than, say, ten years ago – I think of several **elements that can drag people into a whirlpool at the societal and individual level, heightening anxiety and vulnerability.** Might this whirlpool be more causal, the virus more instigational? In my view, most of the effect plays at non-conscious level. Going a bit deeper into them, one can see that each is related to the phenomenon of human attention. One may conclude that there is something deeply wrong with the state of attention.

The following list is incomplete, subjective and exaggerated. One can write a book full of critique and then critique upon this and so on. So, spare me. This is to let you (and me) feel the probability. Also, this doesn't mean that we should avoid all this. We should think about what we are missing.

- Social media enlarging emotional messages x 100
- A.I. means being used to manipulate this even (much) more
- Anxiety from the possibility of being 'liked' or not
- Inundation with 'the latest news'
- Diminishment of people's attention span
- Relative lack of contact with nature
- Stories of dread and doom: global warming, viruses, A.I., ...
- Possibility of complete self-annihilation of humankind
- Mounting stress in general
- Cultural complexity
- Spread of intake of antidepressants
- Advertising: targeting the ego
- Rationalization at work, treating people machine-like
- Computers controlling people almost to the second
- Political manipulation with more sophisticated means
- Choice stress in many domains
- General shortage of true leadership at all levels
- Diminishing trust in truthful news
- Addictions to drugs, food, news, online porn...
- Gamification
- Diminishing sense of deep meaningfulness
- Rampant consumerism, leaving no time for depth

- Artificially induced intolerance of discomfort
- Feeling of alienation from community, even family
- Sanctification of subjective feelings of individuals
- Living from paycheck to paycheck
- More flexible, but superficial relationships
- Feeling like a 'thing' in relationships
- Parental intake of antidepressants
- Children left with little example of profound attention
- Rampant burnout without support from inside out
- Wreaking havoc on the surrounding ecosystem, 'our mother'
- Symptomatic medications: not reaching human depth
- People not dealing with one's suffering inside
- Quickening pace of social changes, no time to adapt
- Older people seeing their world vanishing
- Workers' alienation from product and purpose
- Physicians getting little time to listen to patients
- Mounting administration load for teachers, physicians, etc.

5. What To Do in Times of COVID

March 30, 2020

	Today	Total
Cases worldwide	64.470	790.234
Deaths worldwide	4.162	39.341

[If this text is not your thing, do not comment.]

With a little attentional effort, I start feeling a slight irritation in my bronchi, a little shortness of breath, some pressure in the chest. It's confusing. I can let myself go into this and feel the symptoms even more. Should I consult a physician? That would be me. Well, this does not mean that any symptoms are fake. It just shows how influential the mind can be on bodily symptoms. Research shows again and again that this can also be relevant to (objective) signs, not only to (subjective) symptoms. This indicates that when in acute respiratory distress, it is always important how you orient attention to the symptoms. Likewise, in the following points of advice, what to do lies equally in how you do it. Mechanically following these points is not going to provide their full potential. You have to really mean it.

In general

- Follow guidelines from trusted sources. Don't let any of the ones in this document make you not follow the other ones. I would say: And vice versa as well.

- Note again that *every* infection is mind-body related. Science is unequivocal in this. It's dependent on many circumstances, but mind-body relatedness is always there. Moreover, your immune system is only part of your defense. It's altogether very complex, and your mind is related to it in many complex ways.

If you don't have any symptoms

- Think of the whirlpool image (related to multicausality). It's better to stay out of the whirlpool. [see: "The Message in the Virus"]

- With little effort, you may be doing just the right thing that saves you from being drawn into the whirlpool. Eventually, this small effort may save your life even while it doesn't look so.

- If the news grabs you by the throat, then try to keep yourself emotionally clean. That doesn't mean that you should be emotionless. You may practice the feeling of being sensitive while not being vulnerable. These are two distinct entities. Stated differently: You may care for others while caring for yourself.

- Avoid attention-killers. Too much thumb-scrolling social media may have a negative influence. If you feel it does, restrict yourself to a timeframe.

- Especially avoid feeling panicky while or through being immersed in social media country. If you do, then see yourself as being manipulated by social media mechanisms. It is better to pull yourself out of it and find your inner strength.

- Take care of your body as an integral part of your body-mind. There is only one *you*. You know what to do!

- Take care of your mind. One meditation or guided meditation each day may already be very salutary even while it doesn't look so.

- Smile at everyone you meet outside and, if the occasion arises, practice a little bit of friendly communication from a physical distance. You might compensate for the distance by more social togetherness.

- Stop smoking for a while. Even a few days of non-smoking has a positive effect on your lungs.

- Get enough sleep or deep rest. This by itself also strengthens your immune system at the cellular level, as science shows.

- Contemplate your reasons to be alive and healthy. Even if you 'know' them, your deeper mind likes to be reminded regularly.

- If you get a positive corona-test, remind yourself that this is the time to take it positively and practice what you've just read.

If you have symptoms to a small degree

- Always take them seriously. Do not forego medical consultation.

- Giving deep attention to your symptoms should, at least after a short while, result in a diminishment, small or large. If only a bit, no problem. You are practicing.

- Superficial attention to them may more readily become infested with panicky thoughts (even as non-conscious pre-thoughts) and a heightening of the symptoms.

- Regularly put yourself in an upright position in body and mind as a sign of respect for yourself. If possible, try to stay relaxed. Then try to let yourself become even more relaxed. This is your groundwork upon which you can build further in a better way.

- Practice *slow breathing*. This is not necessarily slow in time. It's more a kind of breathing with attention. Try to follow your breath in its natural flow, even when it's more difficult than otherwise. This way, you 'relax your lungs' and make them more resistant, less vulnerable.

- Picture yourself in a whirlpool, turning around and not getting deeper into it. Try staying relaxed in your imagination. As much as possible, feel your strength. Don't fool yourself. Search *your* strength.

- All in all: relax. Your outlook is brighter when you do so. The more you practice, the more so. It is self-fulfilling to some degree.

- Every symptom, if present to a slight degree, is a defense of your body against the virus. If it doesn't derail, your symptom is your friend.

- Prepare yourself for the eventuality that your symptoms may get worse. Practice the following guidelines, preferably before they are necessary. Rehearse them in order to give to yourself the best you've got inside. Your rehearsals are a sign of your inner strength.

If you have severe symptoms

- This means you are in the whirlpool.

- Don't feel guilty about this. You are not. Moreover, we know that guilt is bad for health in many ways, including immunology.

- At the same time, keep your responsibility for doing the best you can right now.

- Use everything you've got, every second, to also defend yourself mentally.

- You may let yourself be drawn towards a future of health, by that future of health. You can see it as a lifeline to get you out of the present situation. This is especially important at the level of deeper meaning.

- Don't see the virus by itself as the enemy to combat. Your adversary is the whirlpool. The virus is only part of that.

- No matter how deep you're into it, you can get out of it. Never give up. Promise that to yourself. You owe it to yourself. You owe it to others. You owe it to me.

- Every minute you survive, you heighten your chances to get beyond.

- Keep feeling powerful. You may find in yourself a strength that you didn't know before.

- Getting beyond, you may use that power – inner strength – for the rest of your life. You may use it to do something great.

- Deep inside, every person has an 'ocean of deep motivation' to stay alive and accomplish things. It is an infinite ocean. Deep motivation is 'human energy.'

- Your mantra: Stay alive now to accomplish things later.

- You may picture your guardian angel. (S)he is not here to keep you alive but to support you in doing so yourself.

For caregivers

- All the above, of course, are important to you.

- Try to give no less attention to the ones you care for, but indeed less *superficial* attention. Many caregivers (but not all) already know what deep attention means. Now is the time to practice it as much as possible.

- Let your heart be warmed by a smile or a blink of an eye.

- Respect your emotions. Don't let yourself be carried away by them.

- If a patient dies and you have given your deep attention even only during the last few minutes of consciousness, then you have done a very good thing.

- You mean a lot by being you and by doing what you do.

- Give, but don't give yourself away.

- Never give up. Also, never give up another person. A person may slip away but should, especially then, never be 'given up.' This is also crucial for the caregiver's sake.

- It is best to be exceptionally nice to other caregivers and to ask them to be exceptionally nice to you.

- Due to your contacts, you may be especially prone to 'psychological contamination' on the level of profound meaningfulness. You should now and then take special care for this, such as while washing your hands. Relax and also cleanse your 'deeper mind and body.'

6. Rethinking COVID – in the Face of Stress

April 12, 2020

	Today	Total
Cases worldwide	71.756	1.826.022
Deaths worldwide	5.569	119.617

A 'stress' primer

The concept of 'stress' seems simple. Its origin lies in mechanical stress. The way it is mostly used nowadays is also related to a mechanical view on the human being. Many 'stress' tests boil the experience down to a number. Levels of stress are compared to their influence on health and well-being.

To be fully useful, in humans and animals as well, we need a more complex stress-concept, taking into account deeper meaningfulness. I use this more complex concept in this blog, noticing in stress the presence of many self-perpetuating patterns of meaning. One example of deep meaning is <Help, I'm gonna die!>

One doesn't need to be panicky to be stressed. It's all about deeper meaning. Poetry. Therefore, not to be readily analyzed/conceptualized. Therefore, with a simple stress concept, it may be harder to see the correct meaningful correlations. On the other side, with a too broad stress-concept, one risks to use it in an over-explanatory way. This is a scientific challenge.

In stress, as in many other issues, non-conscious mental processing is more important than conscious mental processing. Any 'deep meaning' is first realized at the non-conscious level. Even the stress that one consciously feels is mostly the result of a non-conscious happening. Only from there, we can start to experience anything consciously at all. Only from there also, we can see many influences from mind to body, also in relation to COVID. A proper insight into the importance of non-conscious pattern-based processing is necessary for a proper insight in the importance of body-mind influences, such as in the domain of stress. Unfortunately, that proper insight is generally lacking. This way, the influences may be grandiosely overlooked even when it's a matter of life or death.

In the following, there are knowns and unknowns. I made the text less readable by repeatedly pointing to this. Note, again, that even while 'stress' shows to have an influence, the real influence may be much higher but is unknown since we dearly lack proper insight. Even so.

How we get ill from the virus (probably)

Many people get infected with SARS-CoV-2, which seems to be – **fact** – much more infectious than other coronaviruses. Many of the infected people develop – **fact** – no symptoms or only slight ones.

Within a person, the virus replicates – **fact** – like crazy, making the person a 'virus shedder', especially when at the start of being symptomatic (sneezing, coughing). Thus, almost in every case, the infected person has been able to infect others – **fact** – before he turns very ill.

Stress inhibits – **fact** – a strong immune response. We see this also – **fact** – in the case of vaccination. In COVID, this same phenomenon leads to an even more pronounced viral replication phase. The person develops a huge viral load, becoming a super shedder. That is the opportunity of this virus.

After a weak response, as it often goes, follows a hard one. [see: "Weak, Hard, Strong, Gentle"] In COVID, this shows as a massive immune response, killing viruses but also leading to a huge inflammatory reaction. Here again, stress is a culprit. We know that chronic stress leads – **fact** – to chronic low-grade inflammation. Likewise, acute stress may lead – **fact**

– to intense acute inflammation. An interplay of both makes it especially pronounced. The chronic makes people prone to a massive impact of the acute. Thus, the hard immune response may become life-threatening.

We know that age and anxiety negatively influence the immune response. Both together even more – **fact** – than their simple sum. Thus, older people are more susceptible, get more severely ill, and might also be more infectious, mostly to each other. This may explain – **hypothesis** – the vast toll that we see in homes for the elderly. Once the virus gets hold inside such a home, things may rapidly deteriorate.

Risk factors for a negative progression of COVID are: type-2 diabetes, hypertension, coronary heart disease, smoking. Note that these are also stress-induced conditions. The correlation of these factors with COVID may be the correlation with underlying chronic stress with COVID. Note then again that 'stress' is a very fuzzy concept. Still, it is very important. Look at a cloud (in the sky). A cloud is a fuzzy thing. Yet without clouds, there would be no rain, no plants, nor any complex form of life outside of the oceans.

To do, person-level

Definitely, without the virus, there would not be an immune overreaction against the virus. The measures against viral shedding are mandatory.

At the same time, we should look at the mind. Our mind may be – **hypothesis, which means that we do not know for certain in either way** – at least as important as the virus in being infectious and becoming ill or even dying. Individuals need support in this.

To do, society-level

At the societal level, we need to be careful about how we spread messages and meanings. We want people to keep a distance. 'A bit of panic' may help in this, but at the cost of mounting stress. *Deeply* positive messages are far preferable. Unfortunately, 'deeply' is an orphan in an increasingly superficial world. I see the latter as a saddening fact. My experience over the years is that we are losing depth, which makes many people more and more anxious. [see: "Anxiety"] Older people may be more vulnerable to this, physically and mentally. Knowingly or unknowingly, they experience – **hypothesis** – the trend. They come from another age. More generally, a lack of depth doesn't specifically make those suffer who have a lack of depth themselves. To suffer from it, you need to feel it, to be prone, to be sensitive. Reality in this is highly complex.

Of course, a *deeply* positive message is not just strongly positing so-and-so in the idea that just strongly positing things will – magically? – make them happen. The latter is extremely dangerous. We see strongmen saying so-and-so. At a tipping point of disaster, it backfires enormously. The tragedy becomes complete. The primary victims are vulnerable people. In my view, this may be the essential part of any message: you do it out of care/Compassion for the more vulnerable. In the best case, through this, the vulnerable turn into the efficiently sensitive, which may be the prime reason for Stressional Intelligence.

Indeed: for the more vulnerable in your direct environment and on the other side of town, continent, world. In a global village, everybody comes to the campfire.

We should not denigrate the virus as part of the problem, but it *IS* only part of the problem. Our mind is another part. As said, the non-conscious plays a huge role in stress. The messages should be accordingly.

Looking at the COVID world map

At this moment, weeks into the challenge, it may strike anyone that Europe and the US are hit hardest. India, Africa, and Latin-America are still spared of the worst. However, the virus is gaining terrain. These parts of the world may still fall off the cliff. Or they may not. It remains noteworthy that they haven't yet.

We, from the epicenter of the disaster, should avoid pushing them off the cliff by messages of unavoidable doom. Apart from lots of physical support, they need responsibility in body and mind. Are we a good example of the latter?

Back to Wuhan

I don't want to commit 'culture bashing,' but cannot approve of what happens at live markets anywhere. They should be banned. They are bad for animals. They are also bad for the future of humanity!

The animals in the 'live market' are very stressed. Thus, they are extraordinarily infectious to each other. The ones that are infected get immense viral loads. This happens again and again, creating a specific niche for our type of coronavirus (and maybe already for the next one). It learns to take advantage of stress within an organism. It replicates very quickly and jumps to another organism before the present one gets into immunological overdrive. It carves its niche first in stressed-out animals, learning in the course of many viral generations.

Jumping over to humans, it gets its 'aha experience.' Isn't this human creature an exceptionally stressful animal? So, the human cycle begins, and it goes rapidly. Helped by personal transportation, the virus conquers the world in no time.

The rest will be history. There is always a lesson in history. We should learn it now.

7. Corona Crash

April 18, 2020

	Today	Total
Cases worldwide	80.730	2.300.205
Deaths worldwide	6.679	162.992

The virus and us

A virus is the smallest living thing on earth. And in a way, it's not even living. It doesn't replicate. It lets itself be multiplied. A virus is like a string of information caught in some genetic material that needs and forces a living cell to build an in-between physical carrier: the 'virus' as we can see through a microscope. The living cell, whether bacterial, human, or anything, is like an industrial plant to the virus and eventually dies through this process. The multiplied virus jumps to the next cell, and so on. Relatively seen, the physical carrier of genetic information is extremely simple.

Compare it to us. Our physical carrier (body/mind unity) is extremely complex. Normal humans don't see themselves as 'a string of information caught in some genetic material + carrier' that only uses the carrier to replicate this string. We are the masters of the universe.

Yet, at this moment, one type of virus is seen as 'the enemy of humankind.' A war is waged against it. Even some other wars are temporarily suspended in order to wage this one. Kill the virus! Well, of course, it cannot be killed because it's not living. 'Killing' and 'war' are just elements of a metaphor.

Wartime

And that's what I want to talk about. This metaphor may be part of what leads most of all to an ongoing crash and another pending one. The metaphor is part of our mind. We 'wage war,' but there is nothing to wage war against. Everybody wants to get rid of the virus, surely. Hey. Me too. But waging war, in this case as in any other, lives first and foremost in our mind, and it can kill.

It kills thousands, sometimes millions. Take WWI and WWII. Would there have been any world war if waging-war had not been in the minds of many already long before the first shot?

I see many premonitions in the art of the last decades of the 19th century. People couldn't mentally or morally follow the societal changes, technology playing a substantial part. Concretely, look at Gauguin and other painters of that era in Pont Aven. They were trying to point out an internally dissociated society evolving to the brink. Having been in Pont Aven recently, I saw the inevitability of war – back then – a few decades later. Or rather, the inevitability of war if no other direction could be found for the waging-war inside. The painters showed. People didn't listen and still don't.

In many cases, it is anxiety that leads to war. I mean the anxiety that lives in many people in a certain age and (local or even more and more worldwide) culture. One may say that war is a whirlpool in a stream of anxiety. In a way, a war may incorporate a lot of the energy of this stream. To many, the fact of being at war alleviates. One can see that in any war that has been fought historically. Of course, it is never a solution. In the best scenario, it leads to a change that should have been made long ago. Meanwhile, it irreparably breaks many valuable things and makes the world more ugly.

I don't see the 'war against the virus' as an exception to this. For instance, by now, it becomes clear that, unless many people specifically deal with this issue, the economy will be broken in several valuable aspects. There will be less money for what is deeply meaningful. There will be more suffering from a lack of deeper meaning. Unfortunately, through this, there will be even more anxiety, burnout, and all the pain that comes from internal dissociation. Will there also be less beauty? I hope not.

In 'Rethinking COVID,' I defended the hypothesis that the COVID virus is specialized in taking a stressed-out organism as its industrial plant for multiplication. It doesn't matter to the virus whether this is the master of the universe. As I explained, after a weak response to the virus, the human's defense system goes in full war mode, killing the virus and, while doing so, in regretfully many instances – and each one is of course extremely regretful – also destroying the plant. The human dies through an overshoot of immunological and inflammatory war-waging.

From war to fighting-for

In human mind-body-oneness reality, the physical and the psychological war-waging are not two separate things. They certainly overlap. In my view, they overlap to a significant degree.

> The title of this set of articles was at first 'Mind over COVID.' I got feedback from several readers that this could be interpreted as giving more weight to the mind than to the virus. Especially deeper-mind-negating medical colleagues could see this as hmm, well, what? Preposterous, and worse. First, I was advised to stop thinking aloud, which I didn't. Then I was advised to rephrase and make more palatable, which I did, with pleasure and gratitude.

We are living in a war zone. We wage war against the virus. In a war, everyone is either friend or foe. With only two sides, A and B, it's simple: NOT-A = B. No time for nuance. No room for a broader view. The only way is forward. In times of stress, people tend to think in 'fight or flight.' We want to fight the virus. We take our flight in sheltering at home, in social distancing. These are rational things to do, indeed. But the war metaphor is not rationally straightforward. We need to be wary of that. It can make us act foolishly. It can make us not see what we are fighting against, which may include ourselves.

> Wow, dangerous to say such a thing in wartime. So, we are the enemy ourselves? NOT-B = A? Do I dare to show my face after this?

The main sorry thing that is happening is that, for a long time already, we are *continuously* living in a war zone. Now it's the virus. The metaphor is much broader. It may be anything or anyone. If the war-waging comes first, the enemy is whatever. Where the war-waging comes from is another complex story. It is related to who we are as a species, and even as a living organism. The main thing is that war is never necessary. Yes, we should defend ourselves. Yes, anyone should personally defend oneself. Yes, I dare show my face and will defend it. But war comes with losing rationality. It's the wrong metaphor and has dire consequences.

Fighting-for is not aggression. You can fight for health, for happiness, for life, and all positive things for yourself and others. Fighting-for is not aggression. Fighting-against is. In *Your Mind as Cure*, I start by showing that modern Western medicine is a medicine of war. The enemy is the disease. That may be correct – although still unnecessary – in case of purely physical disease. In psycho-somatic health issues, however, it is the wrong metaphor. Before you know it, the enemy is yourself. Then what? Going forward with no broader view?

On the edge of a precipice, forward leads to crash. At the individual level, forward may lead to death through immunological overshoot. At the societal level, forward may lead to a social, economic, political, and even religious crash. As it happens, this does not need to be an immediate consequence. It may take a while. A whole society may get into a post-traumatic stress syndrome that is like a whirlpool by itself. We should be cautious about this.

> Am I fearmongering now? I don't mean to. I show a dangerous whirlpool and a way out. Also at the societal level.

Many people wage many different wars. We see now several voices already waging their wars, or putting them more at the forefront, towards a post-corona era in which this-or-that, in war-terms. A bas l'infâme! The end of xxx! Whatever. It's just the same war-waging metaphor, with the same 'either A or B' phenomenon. War is never OK.

Moreover, war is not necessary. Its energy is natural. Its form is weird, irrational and inhumane. We should not ever wage war. We should defend ourselves. And we should know ourselves. To do the former well, the latter is essential. Of course, as 'masters of the universe,' we shouldn't expect it to be easy. In *The Journey towards Compassionate A.I.*, I made an effort to contribute.

War is never OK. With a good view of where the energy comes from, we can use it better. Not destructively. Constructively. That is a double gain. In every human matter, this can be brought to bear many fruits.

"So much theory," you might say, but this is a bucket to be filled. After being filled with insight and, yes, personal growth, it starts overflowing by itself. What is supposed to take a considerable effort is effortless. The real effort comes before.

But that is a different story.

Filling the bucket, the bucket itself gets filled with something. Looking closer to what this may be, one can see it is Compassion. Humanity will thrive on this if we get to this. Compassion is not the kind of peace that leads to the next war. It's much deeper than that. It's depth itself. It's poetry.

8. COVID Whirlpool

April 27, 2020

	Today	Total
Cases worldwide	69.621	3.026.613
Deaths worldwide	4.513	214.894

Whirlpool phenomenon

I expand upon an idea about what happens to a person getting more and more COVID symptoms towards a whirlpool that may become fatal.

A *whirlpool scenario* probably happens in many cases of illness. It corresponds with complexity and multi-causal thinking. In crash-course: put many elements together, add more and more 'energy' in the process. You dynamically see a new structure appear that is still based upon the existing elements, yet cannot be *tractably* reduced to them. What happens in the new structure is too complex. There is no magic involved and yet, in practice, it cannot be traced. It can only be theoretically understood, not in practical details. An example is the weather. A whirlwind is close to the image itself. With more energy (a warmer world) we may see more and more whirlwinds.

Humans, and life in general, are another example of complex systems. Continuously, many elements come together and form who we are in body and mind. No magic involved. The 'energy' that is being put in our system is our motivation to carry on, do stuff; in short: live. Our body is extremely complex; our mind – if you want – even more.

> I see 'complex' in the human case always as Open, I have written extensively about the human being as an Open-complex system in *The Journey Towards Compassionate A.I.* In my view, really

intelligent A.I. will also be Open-complex. It's good to know who we are, what A.I. can be, and why it matters. An Open-complex system is Open to its inside as well as to the outside.

So, many elements come together. Our body might seem simple, a set of organs with clear interactions between them like the parts of a car or even an airplane. That may be complicated, but not complex. It is tractable. An engineer may make one. It is mechanical.

Not so with an organic entity, an organism. Organic = complex, not practically traceable. Western medicine is built upon non-complex, Newtonian notions of physics: the universe as a clock, the human being as a clock with distinct parts and a non-complex possible understanding of them. Medical specialists know ever more about ever less. Parts and subparts are seen like those of an airplane. The system is but the sum of subsystems. When there is a disease, you have to look for the broken subpart and repair or replace it.

This may lead to a lot of reproducible fixing and mending. It leads to a lot of products that can be mass-produced and marketed. Business opportunities abound. That way, it is successful – as business. As far as it corresponds to reality, it is also successful in helping the sick and broken.

But it is not the whole reality. Organic reality is at first place complex. Within this complexity, whirlpools lead to illness. Reality is also always multi-causal. The mind is always involved to some degree. In many cases, we have little idea as to what degree. It cannot be put in a box. Contrary to this, the non-complex is like what one can, indeed, put in a box. That box is part of reality, not vice versa. Indeed, it may be a crucial part of reality. It should be respected and used as such. It should not be confused with the whole.

Towards being fully applicable in the organic case, the whirlpool as an image lacks something essential. In a whirlpool of water or air, the individual elements do no augment each other. The energy of the system comes directly from outside. In an organic system, elements may enter a whirlpool and at the same time also energize it in vicious circles or 'self-perpetuating patterns.' The organism can get stuck in such a whirlpool of patterns. The energy 'life' is what comes from several of these elements.

An organism is generally full of feedback-loops. In health, these generally work to attain goals of homeostasis (equilibrium) and allostasis (searching a new equilibrium through change). When feedback-loops become feed-forward, a whirlpool is born. When this passes the borders of health, there is a risk of disease.

Whirlpool and COVID

COVID is a disease caused not by a virus but by a whirlpool. The virus is an element of which we know increasingly more. The mind is another element – or set of elements – of which we still know little. But we do know important directions. Some of them are particularly relevant in the case of COVID, not as 'byproducts' but essential elements in a causal whirlpool:

- stress on inflammation
- anxiety
- hostility
- depression, helplessness
- social isolation, loneliness
- lack of sleep, insomnia
- post-traumatic stress

One can see sub-whirlpools in any of these. All together, one may see a whirlpool of whirlpools strong enough to have a huge nocebo effect. The virus is viral and so is the 'hysteria' acting out at a subconceptual level. Hysteria is close to chaos and so is complexity, so is the whirlpool. It looks like complete chaos in intractability. The consequence, as we see, may be clear and with distinct endpoints.

In a prior article, I depicted the COVID-virus as a stress-virus that has (hypothetically) found its niche in stressed-out organisms. Fitting in this hypothesis is that the virus acts quickly. It exchanges strength for speed within a person and between people. It takes advantage of a whirlpool of acute upon chronic stress, immunological responses (too little, then too late and too much), increased inflammation and cell death, coughing and further cell damage, and the virus itself. Note that the immunological reduction in the first phase, exacerbated by chronic stress, co-creates the niche. In the case of COVID-19, a whirlpool may also be seen as present over an entire population, spreading global hysteria and a lot of chronic stress. The factors just described form further parts. In this, the virus finds its niche of replication. Meanwhile, an acute whirlpool within each individual can quickly go in overdrive but by which time the virus has done what it needs: get on to the next organism. This might also mean that the virus may strike again in the same chronically stressed person. Before the immune defense is built up, it has again done what it needs.

COVID is a case. What we see here – at least with open eyes – is pertinent to many domains in health and healing, such as myocardial infarction, stomach ulcers, migraine, NEPS (kind of psychogenic seizures), all kinds of chronic pain syndromes, tinnitus, allergies, autoimmune disorders.

Implication towards management

Also towards proper management, the whirlpool as an image is relevant in any of these domains. This is where the psyche is probably relevant in the whole of human health and healing. As said: not conceptually traceable. When psychotherapy starts from the traceable, it may be even further away from reality as is a purely somatic attempt of putting it all in a box. Sending a patient from a soma-box (the body, somatic medicine) to a psyche-box (the mind, psychotherapy) in many cases ends with the first box and with no avail. This additionally diminishes 'mind' in the minds of physicians and patients. At least, the soma-box is concrete.

Give to the body what pertains to the body; to the mind what pertains to the mind. The mind doesn't come first to the body, nor vice versa. In COVID, properly taking care of the mind is crucial. However, it should be done in the domain of complexity. In an engineering way, this may seem irrelevant. It is more an art than a merely-engineering. In fact, it is both.

It's special. Denying the art, one may end up with bad quality products and services. This concerns policies, communications, and ways to individually help people.

To this end, I made specific guided meditation sessions to be used in situations of acute stress in which symptoms and other causal elements are playing together. I put these sessions on a user-friendly app et voilà. At the time of writing, there are a lot of acute stress situations for which this app is applicable: people confined to their homes and who suffer from mental issues, patients who are diagnosed or even hospitalized with COVID, their relatives at home with lots of worries, and not in the least: caregivers under extraordinary pressure. I think the whirlpool imagery is applicable to all of them. The – free – app will also be useful in other circumstances of 'acute stress' in the future. Of course, this is also an appropriate, though heartbreaking, entry for 'Compassionate A.I.' which may be built stepwise into the app.

Let's just hope it will reach many.

9. Worst Case COVID

May 2, 2020

	Today	Total
Cases worldwide	**83.127**	**3.446.959**
Deaths worldwide	**5.224**	**244.836**

Right

Is this worst case the future? I would go as far as saying that it is not an impossibility.

Please don't read this text if you are weak at heart.

Numbers

Vaccination is still far away. Experts talk about at least a year before the population can be vaccinated in sufficient numbers to call it a go. A direct cure for COVID is also not evident. Sadly, an empathic wish for a cure will not make one.

The numbers from the labs in several countries show 4-5% of the population being immune at this moment. We need to attain 60-70% for herd immunity as the second option after vaccination. Anyone can calculate that this is 15 x the level we are at now. This makes for a worst-case of eventually 15 x more cases and deaths. The flattening of the curve is not flattening these numbers. We are at the beginning. In Belgium, we see a total of 49.000 cases and 7.700 deaths at present. Before attaining herd immunity and if no vaccine or cure shows up, that means +/- 90.000 deaths in total. Meanwhile, people reach out for a restart of the economy shortly.

Worldwide, there are 240.000 deaths. Of the closed cases, 18% died. That is 7% of all known cases. Curves of total cases and deaths are today [from www.worldometers.info/coronavirus/]:

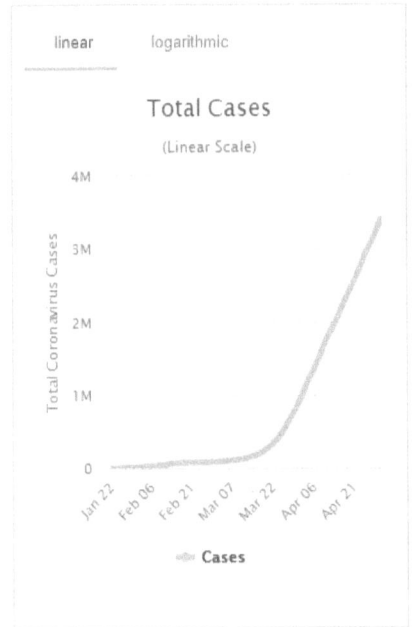

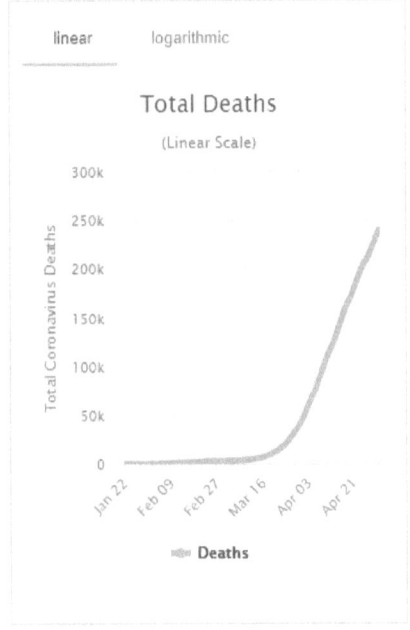

Note the presence of a straight line over the last month. With 3.4 million cases now, we risk going to x 10 or more in numbers of cases and deaths from COVID, worldwide, before vaccination day. Parts of the world are not as infected yet as are Europe and the US. This is not because those people have natural immunity. Latinos and blacks in the US are even more infected and have higher mortality than whites. Since the virus will be with us for a long time, new parts of the world may still become its victims. Due to several factors, the situation may become even worse there. Note that the situation is much worse now in Europe and the US than in China. Who would have thought so two months ago?

According to the Yale School of Public Health, the total COVID mortality may be substantially higher than official numbers are showing. They include people who died because of the epidemic but not from the disease. For instance, being afraid to seek medical treatment for unrelated illnesses. Reported levels of anxiety and depression are rising, which may contribute to increased death from suicide. Probably, the death counts will be revised upward as more reporting comes in. In the UK, the Financial Times estimated twice as many deaths from COVID than official estimates of England and Wales. People may die at home from a pulmonary embolism or heart attack in which the virus plays the role of a catalyst. Pulmonary failure may indirectly lead to failure of other organs, compounded with the result of general inflammation. It's challenging to make an accurate analysis of such cases. Even without direct viral involvement, the stress from the social situation may play a substantial role in much sickness and mortality.

Add to this the collapse of economies, the surge of other diseases through poverty and lack of medical aid in parts of the world, the desperation, violence, etc. We may well be at the very beginning of this too.

Many countries are in lockdown. Some are reopening, but we don't know whether this is sustainable. There is a clear risk of second and third wave after reopening. Many experts are confident in this. The choice seems to be between economic opening and certain surplus death toll, or less opening and economic disaster.

Virology - immunology

There is a huge difference in how people react to viral infestation. Most have little or no symptoms. The young are infected but don't get ill (so much). First to think about is – again – the immune system which is, according to a massive amount of scientific insight, significantly influenced by psychological factors.

Additionally, we don't know how many people are already immune. These numbers appear to be much higher than expected. This shows that, besides the virus, other 'mystery factors' have a significant role to a higher degree than with other viruses. Such factors may be genetics or the psyche.

People who die from COVID generally don't do so because the virus kills too many cells but because of their chaotic immune response. The latter deserves more attention.

We are looking at an enemy outside and how to 'fight or flight.' Vaccination/medication or lockdown/social distancing. This accords to the normal stress response as described in psychosocial literature. More recently, a third response has been added: the coming together and talking. Social togetherness, one way or another. In the COVID case, the stress response may be particularly relevant, given the huge influence of stress on immunology. In another article, I call it the stress virus. It appears to have found a specific niche in stressed organisms. All elements of the enfolding story point to this.

Aftermath

After strong viral episodes from COVID, many get cured. Unfortunately, this is not the end of the mishap to any such person. Among other things, we know little about possible re-infection or even re-infection from inside as with some Herpesviridae leading to zona. 'From inside' in this case means that the virus may be hidden in one's body after the first period of illness. Even after years, it may suddenly reappear. No contact with another infected person is needed.

Due to the high level of inflammation in the lungs, these remain scarred. Look at an inflammation of the skin and scarification afterward. This makes the lungs more vulnerable to several diseases in the future, going from other infections or re-infection with a new corona strain to an elevated risk of cancer.

Viral infections accompanied by strong inflammation are suspected precursors of autoimmune disorders. Multiple sclerosis is one such case. In this, there seems to be an interplay between virus, immune response, and inflammation forming a causal whirlpool. Note that with COVID, we see an extraordinary amount of inflammation. So, the elements are present. Other autoimmune-related disorders are rheumatic arthritis, inflammatory bowel disease, diabetes mellitus, psoriasis, systemic lupus, vitiligo, some thyroid diseases, and so on.

After viral infections, and also related to inflammatory processes caused by them, it is not uncommon to feel depressed or even get into a florid depression. In the COVID case, we already see people with neural symptoms. The virus is suspected to reach the brain in some patients. It is too soon to know the consequences.

More broadly, we may see the appearance of a new viral strain through mutation, another kind of 're-infection' at the social level. The new virus is like a cousin of the previous one. If the cousin is more infectious, even if not more deadly by itself, the chance is that a second wave leads to an even higher fatality at the population level, reaching those who were not infected by the first wave. Improbable? It happened in 1918 with the Spanish flu. The first wave was like a strong typical flu, affecting many people. Then one mutated strand – the cousin – of the virus appeared, being much more deadly than the previous one. People were kept working because of the war effort. Soldiers were displaced en masse for the same reason: war. After four years of war, populations were not in good shape. The stage was set for a second wave that killed, nearing the end of the war, more people in a few months – mainly in September and October of 1918 – than the whole World War itself. And now? 2020. There are four million reported cases. For sure, many more people are infected. There is by far no herd immunity. No vaccine. The virus is not contained. Stress as before. People are put to work again because of the 'war effort,' being at present the economy. I find this immensely dangerous.

So

Of course, it is advisable not to get infected. But within the herd immunity scheme, the statistical risk is unavoidable. In case no more deadly strain appears, one can only hope to be between the 30 to 40% of eventually uninfected people. In the narrowest sense, this is about 'me or you.' The very rich might go and sit on their private islands and wait for herd immunity – or vaccination – then come out again. An insane dystopia.

In my view, the best to-do is to positively boost your own inner defense, including the immune system. Thus, one can diminish inflammation, the risk of dying and of any aftermath and, maybe, also the level of infectiousness, saving time for others towards vaccination day, hopefully somewhere in 2021. There is no magic involved in this. There is no wonder cure. Nevertheless, any immune support is welcome. More generally, inner strength, as is referred to in the last two characters of AURELIS (a project I'm working on for years already).

Scientifically, we know pretty well that the human mind has a significant effect on the immune system. A possible positive effect is evident, although less scientifically investigated in experimental studies, due to the difficulty of organizing such studies. Elements in this difficulty are operational (the study itself), ethical, and financial. Perhaps this time of COVID can enforce a breakthrough in research. At this moment, as far as I can see, there is no sign that this breakthrough is happening.

Us

We are developing tools and are trying to involve financial partners, as well as scientific cooperation to make this possible.

More specifically, we are developing psychological support through an app containing mental exercises and additional how-to and informational background. The app is applicable in any situation of acute stress with a risk to 'drown in a whirlpool of different elements.' One such situation is coronavirus + stress (acute upon chronic and in the broadest sense) + inflammation. Another applicable situation may be that of the caregiver. Even more, a caregiver who gets infected.

This version of the app will be for free for all forever, soon available as the 'Aurelis' app. One can look at it as a key to open the door towards the space beyond. The key by itself may seem irrelevant. Its quality is all-important to reach the goal. This is about subconceptual processing or 'autosuggestion,' the subject of my Ph.D. dissertation and book, and the driving force, in openness, of what lies otherwise hidden behind the placebo effect and empathy. We have a lot of experience with this in many domains. We want to give as much support as possible within the app. With A.I. means, stepwise developing the A.I.-driven coaching chatbot *Lisa*, we can go much further. In this, we have a lot of know-how available, and we also know how to accomplish it effectively. We do lack resources.

As said in the beginning, this text could provoke unnecessary panic. Nevertheless, well, we need to be serious about this, unfortunately; very serious. If you see any way to help, please do.

In short, pointing out:

- The situation is even direr than is generally thought at this moment.

- We entered an era that will last much longer. Also in time, we are at the beginning.

- There is a substantial immunological influence, not only on the amount of people getting ill but also on the degree of illness.

- There is a considerable influence of the psyche on immunology.

- This should be investigated much more deeply and realistically than is the case at present.

- The knowledge that we gain – and already have to a relevant degree – may be brought to bear in practical tools and other means.

We should not fight against the virus but fight for a better future. This includes anything related to this viral disease.

10. Corona Risk

June 6, 2020

	Today	Total
Cases worldwide	**129.632**	**6.990.553**
Deaths worldwide	**4.267**	**402.741**

Today we have these coronavirus curves, worldwide

[from www.worldometers.info/coronavirus]:

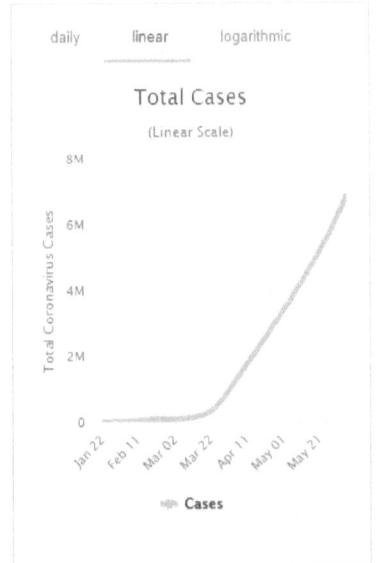

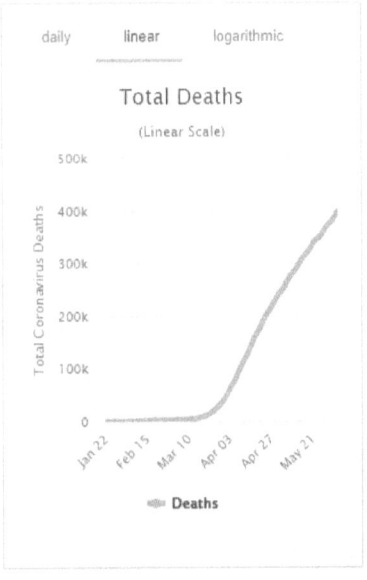

This is not positive. On the 2nd of May (see ' Worst Case COVID'), I was appalled by the linear curve of caseload to that point. Today, it's still linear! The number of deaths per day is slowing down a bit, but not substantially over the last four weeks. We're at +/- 5000 deaths per day worldwide. Including the not officially counted cases, there are probably many more.

In European countries, the numbers are generally falling: many fewer cases and deaths per day. In Belgium, we've come from 300 deaths to 20 deaths daily over the past two months. That is already fantastically good news. As a result, people are going back to the reopened shops, fitness parlors, restaurants, and other public venues. The mental atmosphere is one of relief and exhilaration, with some caution. It feels like coming out of a nightmare. Economically too, we are licking our wounds and trying to recover as if we have escaped the monster for good. We were sinking; now, our children's money is being spent to get us back afloat ASAP. Of course, everybody feels ready to renew economic activity. At the same time, this reopening is going unexpectedly quickly. Most virologists acquiesce, be it reluctantly. We don't know what is happening exactly. Have we lockdowned the virus away or is it something else?

I've never hoped so much to be wrong as I am hoping to be now. What I see in the evolving curves is a negative spiral starting mid-March. I described it back then as a kind of 'hysteria.' In retrospect, more than at the time, this seems a well-chosen term. Hysteria is a phenomenon that happens largely at the subconceptual (mainly non-conscious) level. Conscious control is not a significant factor in this, which is why it is invisible. Not for that, insignificant.

In the way that I saw things happening, the virus pandemic came together with a mental epidemic of hysteria, panic, nocebogenic thoughts: "This is going to be excruciatingly bad." The personal stress and global hysteria played crucial roles in engendering a negative spiral for many, a whirlpool being energized not only by the virus.

In other parts of the world, the disaster is still going on or just starting. Looking at some curves of daily cases until the present:

Daily New Cases in Brazil

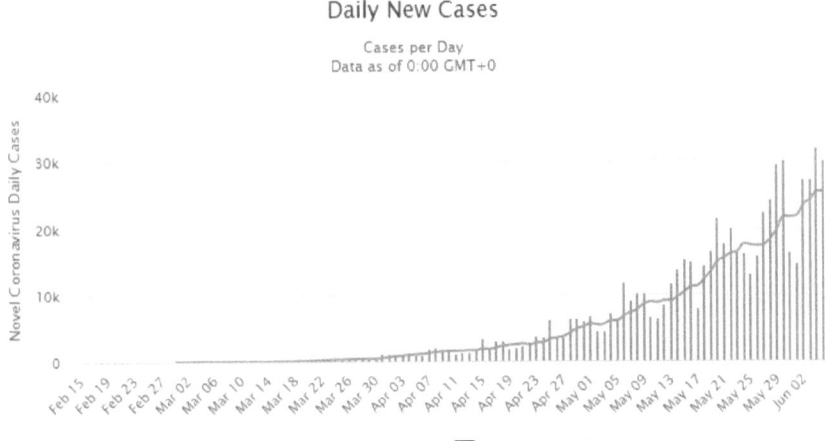

Daily New Cases

Cases per Day
Data as of 0:00 GMT+0

Daily New Cases in Mexico

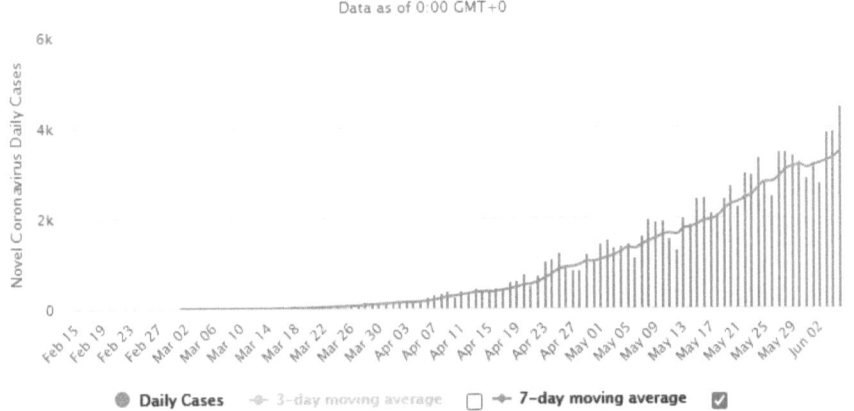

Daily New Cases

Cases per Day
Data as of 0:00 GMT+0

Daily New Cases in India

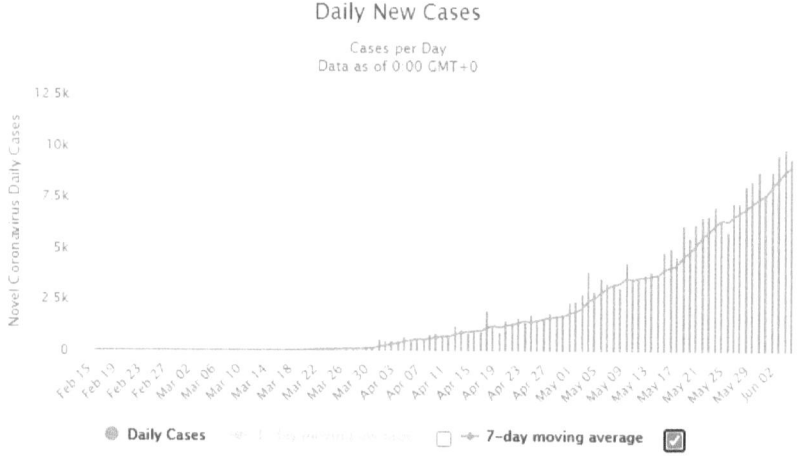

Daily New Cases in Pakistan

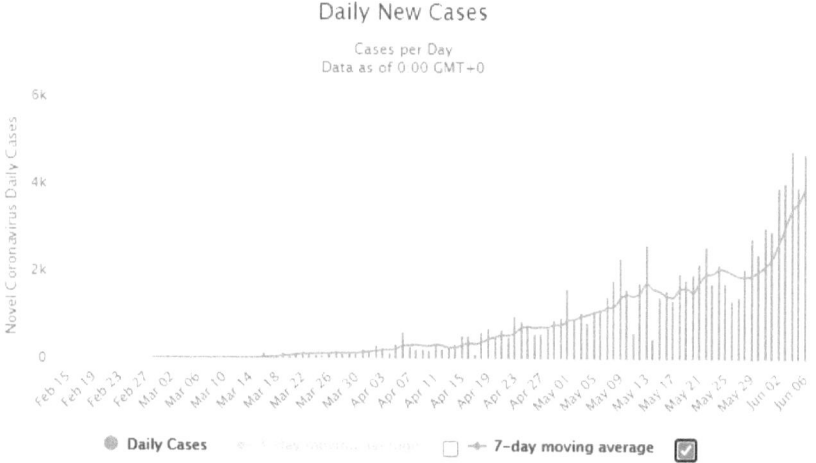

You can see the recurring trend. This looks like the start of a pandemic in these countries. On top of this, these are countries where the actual numbers are probably much higher already. They have no means to keep count of reality as in Europe and the US, nor do they have as much incentive to do so. To be honest, it puzzles me why some parts of the world are lagging behind Europe and the US. One can only see it happening. Also puzzling is Africa: still largely resistant to the virus, although not to a social and economic downturn.

Back to Europe

Borders are reopening. Tourism is promoted almost everywhere on the continent. People feel more and more at ease. Confidence provokes something like the opposite of a negative spiraling. Indeed, we see a positive spiraling, which may be playing according to the same principle as the negative one. Gone is distress (to a considerable degree) and its influence on the immune system. Thus, indeed, the stress-niche of the virus is crumbling. Everybody happy, but the lesson has not been learned. To me, the positive evolution that we are witnessing in Europe at present is an additional strong indication of pending danger. The spiraling may turn back to the other side. Without bad intentions, the media – including social media – may again play a huge role in feeding the whirlpool.

This makes me remember the images from Italy that we saw right before the 'hysteria + pandemia' came hitting with force. As long as the lesson has not been learned, we are at risk of a new and stronger COVID-19 wave. It's like giving a blow with a hammer, then pulling it up to give a second blow.

I'm not writing this to scare anyone without substance. The being scared may have played a big role in the happening. It may also play a significant role in what is to come. Virologists are warning of a second wave in the autumn. We don't know the virus well enough to assume that it will act like Influenza, giving us an intense visit each autumn and winter. If so, then we have two infections at the same time entering our continent and homes. Being different viruses, they may compete between them, but not much. Thus, people may get sick twice at the same time. This also resembles the Spanish flu in the sense that in its second wave, most people succumbed from superinfections.

Meanwhile, herd immunity has not been built against our corona-guest. In Belgium, we are at 6%. Better said, 94% is not immune (some say a bit less). That is almost the total population. Add to this some other unknowns about this specific virus, such as how long people stay immune.

Andrea Ammon, director of the European Centre for Disease Prevention and Control, warns for a second wave in clear terms: "not if but when and how big… people think it's over, which it isn't… it definitely isn't" [www.euractiv.com/section/coronavirus/news/not-if-but-when-european-health-boss-warns-of-virus-second-wave/]

I fear most that we will again get into a negative spiral

This is a whirlpool of *mind + virus* acting in detrimental ways upon the immune system and other physiological defenses, heightening the negative spiraling and starting the same song. On the one hand, there is better protection (masks, instruments, knowledge about the impact of social distancing). On the other hand, the virus may also evolve towards surpassing this protection. As is common in the natural setting, it does so in a brute-force learning over many viral generations. And many generations there are. With each one, viruses may mutate in different directions, including ones that can better take advantage of the niche. Younger people may become targets of infectiousness; the incubation period may prolong; more people may become super-spreaders.

I strongly hope this will not be the case. But we have a history of such, some 100 years ago. The Spanish flu was extremely deadly (10-100 million people) only in its second wave, in the autumn of 1918, after a relatively mild first wave in the spring of that year. The second wave came from a mutated virus. The more people get infected now, the more chance we have to see such a mutation happening.

The lesson that we should learn – in any case – is a lesson about ourselves. We are nature, and we are very complex beings. That is a strength and a weakness. If we learn to deal with it better, we can flip the balance more to the former. Otherwise, before the end of this year, there will again be many more deaths than need be. Plus: What about the economy if the second wave hits us as hard or harder than the first one? It is not possible to keep pouring trillions of dollars and euros in keeping businesses and people afloat.

Thus, the next hysteria-fed whirlpool may be even way more pronounced in that near future. A bit further ahead, a next stress-niched coronavirus may come to haunt us. Actually, the question is not 'if' but 'when.' Will the lesson have been learned? Will humanity be better prepared? We have an opportunity now to diminish also future disaster.

I don't want to scare anyone just for diversion. We are at a moment when things can turn out very badly in a way that only some living humans have seen before. At least, we should examine this from every possible angle. I don't see it happening.

In conclusion: The absence of mind in COVID-19 causal thinking is costing many lives. It may cost many more even by the end of this year. I am urging appropriate research AND action at the highest level. It would be devastating to see the need for this only in retrospect.

The future

Well, mainly in a few months already. Since I don't have a crystal ball, this comes from intuition, rational thinking, a whole lot of research, and experience.

Until the miracle vaccine is developed, this virus will stay present on the planet, going up and down in different areas. The economy will drive individuals and groups to persistent risk-taking behavior.

In Europe and the US, autumn will come with an influenza epidemic like every year. This year will combine the influenza season with a resurgence of corona, and with the risk of hysteria resurgence. If the latter enters the picture profoundly, there will be a renewed whirlpool phenomenon in many individuals and society. Another lockdown may be specifically postponed for economic reasons, at least in several areas, adding to the whirlpool: heightening the risk of an even more severe lockdown and economic downturn, people becoming more and more aggressive to one another about core values (immediate life versus money and the future, race-related factors). Politically, the doors will be ajar towards some forms of 'very tough leadership.' Something 'like we have never seen before' in many decades?

In the US, the numbers of daily new cases and deaths are past a peak. Interestingly, the numbers are increasing in some states, decreasing in others, while experts do not know why. Might there be nocebogenic factors at play, invisible unless you use the right mind-o-scope? Meanwhile, people become demotivated and more careless about social distancing. In my view, it's not so much the carelessness which will provoke the next peak as will the renewed 'hysteria' on top when numbers start rising again in seemingly uncontrollable ways.

The damage will be least in the socially most prudent cultures (China, Japan, South-Korea). Apart from and much deeper than any political system, this is probably mainly related to people having relatively and generally seen a basic trust in how most other people will act to the benefit of society. Compare this to the much more individualistic West. Today, I was walking over the Groenplaats in Antwerp, Belgium. There were a lot of people laughing, sitting on terraces drinking and shouting without face masks. Then one person struck me wearing a mask. It was an Asian woman. To me, this one woman says it all. So, am I a racist if I have more esteem for Asians in this regard than for people as white as myself? Today, China is in the news with a pocket of 57 new cases. At the same day, the US gets 25.300 new cases and Las Vegas booms again.

In the poorest areas of the world (much of the underbelly), there is no way this virus will stop anytime soon. Look at a combination of the necessity of people going to work with an impossibility to protect themselves. This happens within an environment of additional risk factors, such as protein deficiencies, and the lack of medication for superinfections.

Worldwide, the number of daily new cases is still going up. Fortunately, the number of daily deaths is past a peak and rather stabilized over the last month. However, several very populated countries with poor healthcare for most inhabitants are seeing an increase of daily deaths.

One can foresee catastrophic developments in deaths, economic downturns in those countries, and other related catastrophes in view of sheer numbers. Sorry for the bad news.

The biggest risk is a virus mutation into an even more human-unfriendly form...

...especially if that comes with less human immunity for that specific mutation. Of course, at the individual virus-level, the risk is infinitesimally small. But there are many viruses. Each new infection – in any person in any country all over the world; remember how it all started with one human infection – adds to the risk. The 7.5 million known cases of human COVID-19 at present, of which half are still active, are ominous. This is one crucial element in the competition between virus and humanity. Thus, several factors are reminders of 1918. This may seem far-fetched until it happens. At least, the risk is real. What shall we do?

Meanwhile, the race is not simply between the virus and conceptual thinking: face masks, social distancing, lockdown, virus-blockers, vaccines. The race includes – and will be mostly determined by – subconceptual thinking: the so invisible meaning-level that defines our humanity in many ways. At other places, I have written extensively about it as our 'basic cognitive illusion.' It is the only important level given any definition of 'importance' itself. In the few months and years to come, it will be central to the existence of millions and the wellbeing of billions.

I mean, virus-related.

After that comes the next challenge.

11. Summer of COVID

June 13, 2020

	Today	Total
Cases worldwide	134.982	7.889.692
Deaths worldwide	4.238	433.066

It's almost summer in Europe. COVID-19 seems to be a recent nightmare. Glad it's over. But it isn't, of course.

There are several ways in which it isn't over:

- A second wave will probably hit Europe and the US in the autumn. It may be even much worse, given the pandemic of a century ago.

- Worldwide, the number of daily reported cases is still increasing week after week.

- COVID-19 is raging in other parts of the world. The disaster there may become much more prominent than in the more economically developed world.

- Other coronaviruses are probably finding their way to the same niche: stressful organisms, including us.

- We cannot exclude the possibility of a mutation of the virus that will make it more dangerous. See Spanish flu, 1918, death toll: 10-100 million.

- Part of the problem is the economic downfall: countries on the verge of collapse due to the first wave cannot take another blow. This may have huge secondary effects, such as populations getting on the move, especially with climate change as an accompanying disaster.

- An even more essential part of the situation is that this is about us, about the human being in general. Many illnesses are of the mind rather than exclusively the body. In COVID-19, the mind is being ignored in a truly insane way. That's a pity. Seeing the mind in this issue may open eyes to its influence on many other matters, which are even more significant than COVID. Yes, I mean it when I write it.

The COVID-19 adventure may pass an entire planet without being taken as a wake-up call. At this moment, almost nowhere is the mind discussed as a potential element in the whirlpool. We now have a European summer as a resting point. That only lasts three months. Of course, other parts of the world don't have this resting point, on the contrary! Let's not wait.

Europe thinks it has been smart and (+/-) disciplined, so, virus (+/-) gone. A triumph of science? But the reality is very different from the show. We need science indeed, much more than we presently have. We need more rationality and, at the same time, more depth.

A coronavirus is different from an influenza-virus. But some common cold viruses are also of the corona type. We can look at the science about this. Interestingly, the influence of stress on common cold was investigated and proven already 30 years ago [Cohen et al., 1991]. This brings us eerily close to COVID-19.

Is the COVID-19 virus then no more dangerous than a regular flu virus? Hah, politically hazardous question. One can already hear knives being sharpened. Will he dare to write the unsayable? Well, no. COVID-19 is more dangerous than the flu. But if you could really take the whirlpool out of the picture, the difference might become substantially smaller. If, on top of this, one could use one's mind in optimal ways, then I cannot confidently say that the difference would be significant. But since we are not there, the difference is clearly present. There is no denigration meant in this. It's an admonition. What else can I say? Use your mind as a cure. Combine it with every other means at your disposition.

Seasonality

> "Whoever wishes to investigate medicine properly should proceed thus: in the first place to consider the seasons of the year..." *Hippocrates (circa 400BC)*

Note that symptoms of the common cold usually appear in autumn and winter. In May and during summertime, common colds are rare. We see, accordingly, a diminishment of COVID-19 in 'common cold countries.' Probably, we have been lucky that the pandemic took off only in March/April, almost at the end of the influenza season. So, we may ask, have we indeed been lucky or is the COVID season constrained to the end-of-winter period? In the autumn, will the COVID-season show to be just displaced in time or is it more extensive than the influenza period? Will it show its full-blown presence from October till April? Will we have more deaths from corona than from influenza every year, even with vaccination? Those are some of the many things that we don't know yet.

Do we win the 'battle against influenza' every year? No, the time of the year does it for us, until autumn strikes again. Experts are not unanimously convinced that this seasonality, as in the case of influenza, is mainly virus-related. Another hypothesis is that the observed seasonality of influenza is the result rather of a constant level of infection mediated differently by the host immune system over time. People may be susceptible to infection at different times of the year by pathogens which are present year-round. [Dowell SF., 2001] Complex networks of interactions among patients' immune systems, society as a whole, weather conditions, and the continual adaptation of viral antigens to form new strains are probably responsible for seasonal flu infections. The elucidation of all this is by far not finished. A lot remains unexplained. Will the explanatory holes be filled rather by body or mind? Am I suggesting something inappropriate?

One thing is sure: the seasonal trend of some viruses is very sharp. See this curve from www.cdc.gov/flu/about/season/flu-season.htm :

Peak Month of Flu Activity
1982-1983 through 2017-2018

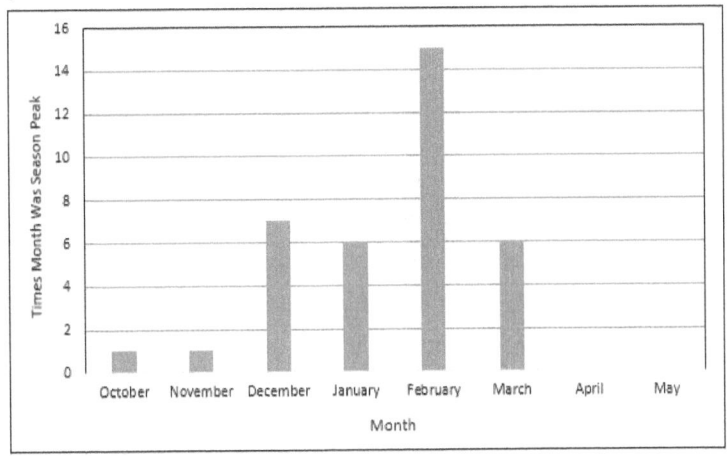

This is in the US, without influenza lockdown, nor social distancing and face masks. Note the disappearance in the summer and re-appearance in autumn-winter. Several other respiratory viruses also circulate during the flu season. Note that affective disorders can also be seasonal. [Kurlansik et al., 2012] Different parts of the world show different curves of viral infection. In some, there are no peaks but year-round activity.

Corona is different, but not that much. For instance, a recent study by the University of Michigan School of Public Health tracked a group of participants (varying from 900 to 1440 subjects) over 8 years, looking at the prevalence of the four most common human coronaviruses in the population. They concluded that coronaviruses are sharply seasonal, appearing to have similar transmission potential to influenza A in the same population. [Monto et al., 2020] The authors noted a peak aggregate month of all four coronaviruses between January and February. One of the four similar curves:

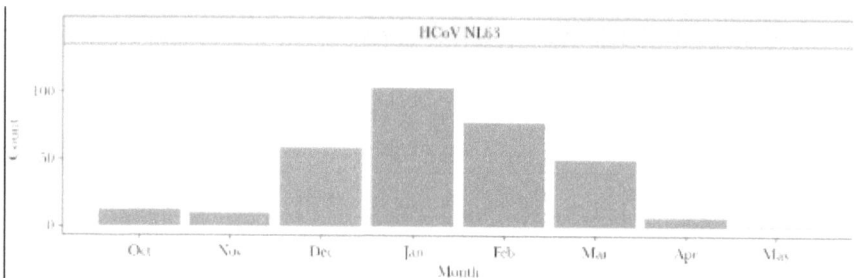

Other and prior studies have corroborated these results. [Killerby et al., 2018] This should not be confounded with common colds from several other viruses that may be present throughout the year. We are dealing specifically with a coronavirus now. Moreover, SARS-CoV-1 was also linked to climate conditions (mainly cool and dry areas). MERS-virus, at least in lab circumstances, also appears to behave in a season-dependent way.

Laboratory experiments demonstrate that temperature and humidity affect the stability and viability of coronaviruses and influenza, including SARS-CoV-1 [Chan et al., 2011] and SARS-CoV-2 [van Doremalen et al., 2020]. This includes the inactivation in tissue culture over 14 days with differences from slight at 4°C to complete at 22°C. [Chin et al., 2020] "*This is thought to be due to changes in essential viral outer proteins and lipids as well as droplet matrices during droplet, and fomite transmission. For example, environments with lower relative humidity may lead to droplet evaporation and smaller droplet sizes. This affects how fat virus-containing droplets travel through the air and where they deposit in the airways.*" [Kanzawa et al., 2020] 'Fomite' is any inanimate, contaminated object.

"The first two major waves of weekly laboratory confirmations of MERS-CoV cases closely followed the seasonal epidemic waves of influenza A in the Middle East." [He et al., 2015] The previous SARS outbreak in China, as well as the present one, occurred in cold, dry wintertime [Sun et al., 2020], probably due to conducive environmental conditions for prolonged viral survival in bats and humans.

To be precise, this does not mean that a 'seasonal' virus does not appear out of its preferred time of the year. Nature is seldom black or white. Of course, viruses that peak at specific periods every year are also present throughout the year. People may get infested all over the year but without getting ill, or just slightly, or only a few people get it. They get a bit of flu. They may get a secondary infection by bacteria and the diagnosis of bacterial pneumonia. They die of old age. In these cases, the virus does not really show itself, unless, of course, it provokes a severe outbreak such as we see now with COVID in different regions of the world. These outbreaks do not show that the new coronavirus is not seasonal. The seasonality comes on top of the hiccups, large or small. In this sense, the present situation in the US is hugely alarming. The whirlpool roars even out of season. It may be that air conditioners are acting a bit as season-simulators. This could be investigated epidemiologically.

In conclusion, we may say that the score for corona seasonality until now is 6-0 in favor of seasonality. About COVID, we don't precisely know yet, but there is no argument for it to be an exception. In the meantime, we have to make heartbreaking decisions. Of course, this perplexes me more than anything about the mind not being taken seriously. Shouldn't we investigate anything with even the slightest glimmer of hope for relief? On the other hand, this is not at all a 'slight glimmer.' This is of utmost seriousness!

That shows, into the unknown, a strong probability of asynchronous seasonal global outbreaks with in the tropics a more year-round persistence, whether or not in its disastrous guise. This may be part of the explanation for the high prevalence in Brazil right now. Africa remains an enigma.

As to Australia, South-Africa, and Santiago de Chile, these are three places of wintertime when the Northern hemisphere enjoys the summer, that is, more or less now at the time of adding this little paragraph. We see much COVID, but no absolute disaster. So, will things turn out not-too-bad in European and US winter? While there is enough uncertainty to keep hoping, looking at the climate in those three regions, temperatures are striking. Those are not winters like ours. One can compare their winters with our months of April. That's when our corona season ends every year. Coronaviruses seem to love 5°C or less. Southern winters in the three mentioned regions witness averages of 10-14°C. Factors such as humidity and UV light also play a role. We seem to be living in the preferred combination for our little guests, in wintertime. Not in summertime.

The point is that we did not win this battle.

Let alone the war, even though it may appear so at present, and we have been given this impression more or less. Experts should not be chest-pounding (as many of them aren't). To be honest, economic reasons also seem to play a significant role in how people in Europe are led to be confident that the worst is over. If so, then it would be misguided and short-sighted. Virologists especially can warn people more openly for a second wave, be it a big one or several smaller ones. It matters a lot for many people and businesses to know about this, even to know the uncertainties. In a few months from now till then, money can be spent differently, more wisely, with this knowledge. But it is a politically tricky statement with a huge counterfactual risk involved. If speaking out the full risk helps towards more caution, few people compare with the deadlier alternative. If part of the – even well-considered – gamble turns out badly, everybody indignantly knows. Here, true leadership is needed. This is what it's for. May I refer to my book about Open Leadership?

Brazil now has a coronavirus death toll of 42,720 fatalities, second only to the US. I take Brazil as an example of what happens in many other countries of Latin-America and more. We saw a Brazilian curve in a previous chapter. Let's look at Egypt today as just another example (from www.worldometers.info/coronavirus):

Daily New Cases in Egypt

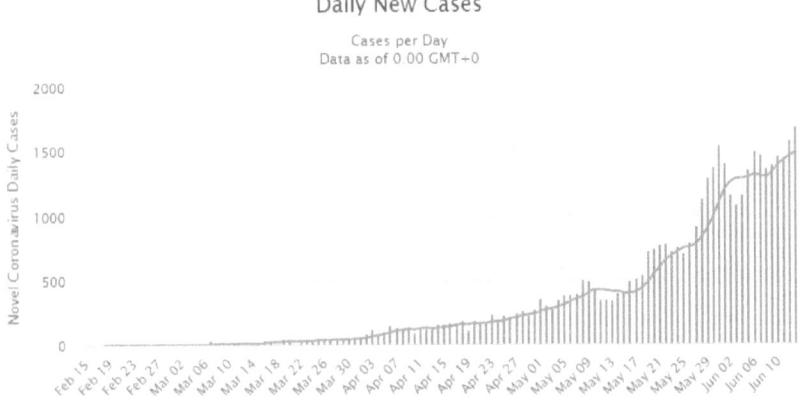

So, in Brazil, with its hotter temperatures, it may be surprising that so many deaths are to be deployed, and given challenges of reporting, probably many more. Does that contradict seasonal influence and, thus, the idea of pending return in Europe + US in a few months?

Unfortunately not. As said, warmth is not the only relevant issue in seasonality. A complex interplay of factors is responsible. In Brazil, we see an influenza season that peaks in June till August, plummeting in September. As said, corona is not influenza, but it's not very much different in behavior (droplet-mode of infection). In this sense, it's not surprising that it is surging now. The odds are that COVID-19 will be ravaging through the land till September. If it plummets then, we have another clear admonition to brace ourselves in Europe + the US, as the viral momentum will be regained in reverse to the South.

Lockdowns

Has the first lockdown in many countries been for naught? Good question. I think the answer is 'no.' But lockdown comes at such a terrible price emotionally and economically — which is also health-related in several ways — that things may not be clear-cut. Responsible politicians have a difficult job of calibration. If they are truly responsible, we should be lenient to their mistakes. We should not ask for their omniscience, but only for their sincere commitment. The lockdown has not been for naught, but with more openness, it could have had a much better effect on people and businesses. I ask for a commitment to look into the matter from every possible angle.

My advice for the next period of possible lockdown is not to use panic as a means to make people cautious. Panic doesn't last, and it creates whirlpool-energy. Don't treat people like puppets on strings because that way, you make them into puppets on strings. They may become resentful afterward. Also, those who are by nature not prone to hanging on strings get a hard time being true to themselves. They may try to bring more common sense but − through the puppet-making − encounter much resistance. This way, decent voices get subdued and make way to populist messages. That's not what anyone profoundly wants.

In case of a second wave, we have − hopefully − the incentive of social distancing, face masks, respirators in place, experience in ICU, and hopefully some effective medication. Nevertheless, if people get into a whirlpool of hysteria again, this may again necessitate a lockdown. There will again be many infections and deaths because probably again, the lockdown will come too late (in the West). There will again be a huge burden to healthcare workers. Will there again be white cloths of support hanging from windows? Super, but even better would be an avoidance of a considerable part of the disaster.

It is clear to me that, without proper subconceptual support, panic will strike again and with renewed vigor in Europe and the US after the summer. Having a clear idea about what has happened recently and may happen again rather soon (the whirlpool) can relieve the damage not with a factor 0.1, but, in my view, with a factor 10. That is said as quickly as anything. Clear insight is crucial.

Of equal importance is the way of communicating this. The recent past doesn't make it easier. Lots of people have died with the primary cure being present − but not reachable − inside themselves. How sad can it be?

>I can only say that I've tried − not well enough − to make it open, to 'promote' for instance my recently published book *Your Mind*

as Cure. This will haunt me for the rest of my life; thank you very much. I received a fair amount of backlash and negation. In view of my credentials in several domains, I think I'm not less scientific than any of my medical colleagues. Many prefer zero-tolerance in personal risk. It is, of course, never too late for this.

So, how to communicate this in a world that is caught in a basic cognitive illusion of not-seeing one's depth and its influence on many things? The difficulty lies in how to combine an admonition to not get panicky with avoiding additional negative emotions of resentment and guilt. Public communicators might take additional coaching-lessons in this.

This does not mean that the conceptual defense (everything that is now regarded as to be done against the virus) should be abolished or even diminished. On the contrary, if COVID-19 comes haunting us again, we need to go for the full Monty, and well soon enough. That lesson has been learned once.

It's even more important since a second wave will come with crowds being less motivated to be locked down. The first time, the puppets accepted the strings, having +/- total confidence in experts. The second time, patience may run dry. Expert-distrust may surge. The puppets may cut themselves loose and get into even more whirlpoolian trouble. Then what? I do expect that IF social trust in being able to win 'the battle against COVID' reaches some low point, the whirlpool will become re-enacted. Once it does so, we are in for a complete cycle: draconian measures to rebuild trust. That will – in the if situation – surely happen again, but will trust be restored before May 2021? In non-European/US countries too, the same phenomenon seems to play a substantial role. It may be less, or with a time-lag, but horrible stories reach smartphones everywhere.

Vaccination

Seven billion takes some time. So, who will get it first? The lack of vaccination in poor regions may enhance distrust and become fuel in the whirlpool. Resulting tensions will be felt at all sides. Moreover, people who take influenza vaccine shots at present notice that each year, they need another shot. That's because the flu virus continuously mutates. This coronavirus also mutates continually, hopefully not as quickly. If it doesn't diminish in virulence and fatality rate, then we're in for a very long time.

The general communication about 'final exit' is that this will happen in the way of developing the vaccine, and that's it. Of course, it needs to be made in huge quantities (billions?). We could live with that. But It's not the end of the story. Different viruses, different vaccinations, complications, and effectiveness. There is currently still no vaccine that prevents HIV infection or treats those who have it. Vaccination against former SARS in mice led to pulmonary immunopathology on a challenge with live SARS virus, suggesting hypersensitivity to SARS-CoV components. [Tseng et al., 2012] The same direction has been noted with MERS. [Agrawal et al., 2016] Of course, progress can be made at any time.

Measles vaccination in two doses gives effectiveness of +/- 97%. That would be great to achieve for COVID-19. However, some vaccinations against other viruses are much less effective. A vaccination against COVID-19 will most probably not be like the one against polio, but more like the one against influenza. We will need (expensive) vaccinations again and again.

More troubling, vaccination will not provide total immunity. The general communication appears to be: Being vaccinated makes one safe. It doesn't work that way with every virus and probably also not with this one. It doesn't make you safe, only safer. We may compare with influenza, although it needs to be said that the mutation rate of corona is slower and thus vaccination can be more efficient. It may mean that we don't need a yearly revaccination, but every two or three years. In the influenza case, note that despite an existing (ongoing) vaccination, every year still sees 100.000s of fatalities. Quoting from the Centers for Disease Control and Prevention (www.cdc.gov/flu/vaccines-work/vaccineeffect.htm): "While vaccine effectiveness (VE) can vary, recent studies show that flu vaccination reduces the risk of flu illness by between 40% and 60% among the overall population during seasons when most circulating flu viruses are well-matched to the flu vaccine." From another report (www.cdc.gov/mmwr/volumes/69/wr/mm6907a1.htm): "According to data from the U.S. Influenza Vaccine Effectiveness Network on 4,112 children and adults with acute respiratory illness during October 23, 2019–January 25, 2020, the overall estimated effectiveness of seasonal influenza vaccine for preventing medically attended, laboratory-confirmed influenza virus infection was 45%." So, not 100% but around half of that. This makes a huge difference: many deaths, continuous anxiety, and an ever returning discussion about whether or not to go into lockdown (soon enough). On top of that, every mass vaccination leads to side effect, including some mortality through the vaccination itself. So, to what extent are we going to take this risk by giving it to younger people in order to disproportionately protect the older?

Interestingly with respect to vaccination is also the research about how the mind may affect the efficacy of vaccination against several viruses. [Yang et al., 2002], [Zimmermann et al., 2019], [Godbout et al., 2006] In general, acute stress heightens the response, chronic stress lowers it. What about acute upon chronic stress? Acute versus chronic is a crude distinction. The more relevant distinctions we make, the more the phenomenon of 'stress' appears to be connected. My conclusion is that mind and vaccination are not two separate worlds. Moreover, having the one in place does not make the other unnecessary. We definitely need both.

Second wave?

In terms of the death toll, there is room for a second wave. More than 1.7 billion people have an underlying medical condition putting them at risk of a severe COVID-19 infection.

I argued before that the new coronavirus should be seen as a stress virus. It takes advantage of chronically stressed-out immune systems. Its propensity to provoke a whirlpool is its niche, its way to make some people short spreaders, and spread itself to the next organism. I hypothesize that this virus is a relatively weak one, at the same time, a quick one. It bets on speed, not on strength. It prefers a weak milieu in which it can act rashly.

Its relative weakness may explain why the whirlpool phenomenon can readily diminish in strength. In Europe, over just a few weeks, cases went down, and reopening did not make them rise again until now. Falling numbers make people more confident that they will get even lower. Thus, nocebo diminishes too. Below a tipping point, we are stronger than the virus. But it can also rapidly regain momentum. Below the tipping point, it's rather safe. Once above, things can rapidly deteriorate. The whirlpool is a self-enhancing and self-perpetuating pattern in which the mind should be taken seriously at every level.

Lately, Iran shows that a second wave is possible, probably not as only the result of better testing, but rather of easing the lockdown. The curve of daily cases at 16th of June (from www.worldometers.info/coronavirus), with deaths also rising as expected in the last few days:

Daily New Cases in Iran

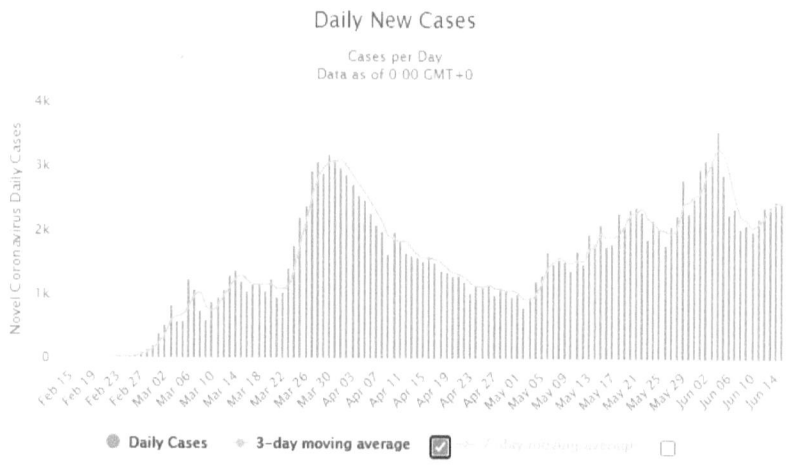

How likely is a huge second wave in Europe and the US in case no wonder drug or procedure would come along? 'Huge' may be defined as: provoking at least as many deaths as until now, despite renewed lockdown and other conceptual measures. That is, with realistic counting, at least a million deaths worldwide, of which 320.000 in Europe+US. Nobody knows, so what are arguments for and against? Listing some:

- Things can quickly drastically change, as seems to have been partly forgotten at present. We just collectively experienced an example that we didn't imagine possible five months ago. The fact that it has happened points to the probability of happening again.

- Other coronaviruses are among the common cold viruses. These show a clear seasonality: little to no presence in the summer, very much in wintertime. Top months are January – February. We have been lucky in 2020 that infections started going at full force only in March - April. Typically, the corona presence is already sharply declining by then.

- Until now, seasonality in other parts of the world is compatible with the prior point.

- Natural herd immunity is still very low at +/- 6%. That is: Almost everyone can still become infected and ill.

- Each year, the common colds reappear with somewhat changed mutated viruses. A one-time immunity is not enough. The present coronavirus is likely to act like other coronaviruses and influenza.

- Immunity to other coronaviruses mostly lasts 6-12 months post-infection. Thus, people who got COVID-19 in the spring might get it again in the autumn or winter.

- Autumn and winter will come with the usual influenza epidemic. COVID will come on top of this with many people weakened by flu.

- More people will start thinking this is with us forever. Many will become depressed and may just 'give up.' Also, they may become less cautious for themselves and others before getting clinically depressed.

- The trust in experts may be much lower next time, making it harder to impose a new lockdown (soon enough). Economic arguments will also be much harsher.

- Vaccination, if and when attained, will probably work at +/- 50% efficacy.

- As to antiviral medication: Hopes are high and realizations are poor until now. There may be a breakthrough.

- There will be no shortage of face masks, hopefully.

- In-hospital mortality has declined over the months for patients with the same symptomatology, due to gathered medical experience.

- China contained the virus through draconian measures that are not possible in the West. Also, a small upsurge in China meets quick and decisive action through local lockdowns. Most probably, Western countries will be too slow.

- The Spanish flu of 1918 showed quite a hefty influenza epidemic in spring. The second wave came in autumn with much more force and mortality than caused by four years of WWI.

- Arguably, the stress levels of many people worldwide will be higher than ever due to social and economic evolutions. Adding to the whirlpool will be (social) media sowing panic about the second wave. Moreover, many people will still suffer from post-traumatic stress from the first wave experiences.

- There's an increasing risk of another coronavirus. There have been three new ones in the last two decades. Before that, there may have been only a few more in two millennia.

Will there be one big second wave or several smaller ones? This will probably depend less on the virus but on our way to handle risks. From mind-perspective, it will depend on how people react. Will there be panic and a feeling of loss of control? Will there be motivation to socially distance and wear face masks? With tourism going on in many places, a resurgence may likely occur at several spots at the same time and the virus can spread quickly. Will we then know in which direction to track? Will people's confidence flip-flop?

After a second wave, people's confidence may be even harder to restore. The expectation upon 'again' may be higher; nocebo more pronounced.

Some experts suggest that a second wave will be less pronounced because a virus weakens with subsequent mutations. It needs hosts to reproduce. Fewer people, fewer hosts for the virus. It does not have as its aim to kill us, but over its generations, to become maximally sustainable. For instance, the influenza A viruses are probably descendants of the Spanish flu virus that ravaged the world in 1918-9 in three (or more) waves. It causes fewer fatalities now just because it needs hosts. The principle is that more fatal ones have less chance to keep reproducing. The competition here is between different strains of viruses. In a sense, we are their battlefield. But like the Spanish flu, a second wave may also be very much stronger. It is possible that back then, people were extremely demotivated to 'go on' in a seemingly endless war, and on top of that, the recurring disease in the months of September and October. The armistice of 11/11/1918 may have been to some degree just another symptom of this massive burnout.

Dexamethasone

Wonder drugs may come along. Hopefully, they do. Just now, dexamethasone is in the news, although not yet in scientific publications, nor have data sets been made available for other researchers to scrutinize. But it seems wonderfully good news indeed. This will probably become part of standard COVID therapy. Worrying may be a side effect of dexamethasone: in certain circumstances, it heightens psychotic delirium. This is a complication with corticosteroids in general. [Kenna et at., 2011] As it happens, patients with severe COVID – when dexamethasone may become most indicated – frequently suffer from altered mental states or delirium, with rates of up to 70% in cases of severe illness. [O'Hanlon et al., 2020] Occasional descriptions are of a kind of prolonged bad trip through taking drugs. Some patients talk of preferring to die. Some need to be restrained. Antipsychotic treatment for hospital delirium shows a lack of efficacy and potential for adverse outcomes. [Nikooie et al., 2019] Non-pharmacological approaches (reorienting communication, early mobilization, therapeutic activities) are difficult to administer in the elderly [Hshieh et al., 2018] and, as a matter of fact, especially in cases of COVID. Also, this doesn't end with getting better physically. In some (many?) cases, it even gets worse when the patient is dismissed from the hospital. Little attention goes to this, but it may be a big problem. One should not only look at the deceased but also at the survivors.

Of course, this or any other wonder drug should not diminish the attention for the mind. In this case, as dexamethasone works through its influence on the immune system, it should even heighten such attention. The whole domain of psychoneuroimmunology shows that the mind and the immune system are very much intertwined. In future proper management of COVID – as in all of medicine – the mind and the body should be seen as the unity they are. One should say: the unity that it is. Looking at the human being as one unity of body and mind brings a much more positive story. For instance, referring to the app that you encounter at the beginning and the end of this book, I see a combination with dexamethasone as more than just a summation of both. On the one hand, within their mental exercises, users can integrate any idea of possible support and use it positively. On the other hand, having used the app and (still?) needing dexamethasone, they may be stronger to deal with a mental whirlpool that could otherwise push them into psychotic delirium.

Meanwhile, new studies are showing the importance of the mind in relation to COVID. One excellent study showed the influence of COVID-related anxiety upon psychosomatic symptoms and disease. This is no surprise. The same influence acts upon the immune system in general, thus also on COVID-progression, closing this cycle in the whirlpool. [Shevlin et al., 2020]

Fortunately, by taking mind seriously, a lot can be done.

But it may take either sufficient investment in software or many human resources. The Aurelis-app 'Acute stress' is one element.

Human depth doesn't cost anything by itself. That's because it is not valued and doesn't come in neat packages. This summer and afterward, it may have the most significant Return On Investment of any time, in human health, lives and the worldwide economy, if we take action in due time.

Which is, of course, as soon as possible. Unfortunately, we haven't learned much from the first wave in respect to mind and COVID.

The curves of June 20 show no reason to be complacent [from www.worldometers.info/coronavirus/] at 464.000 deaths:

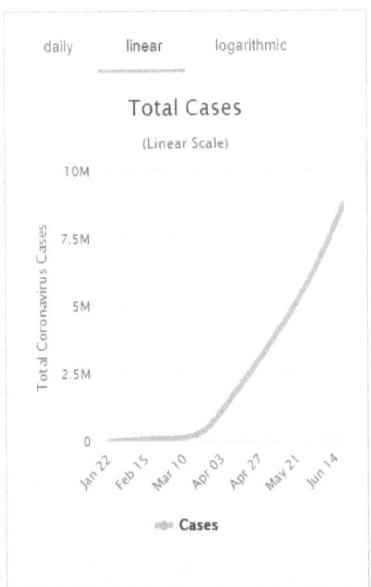 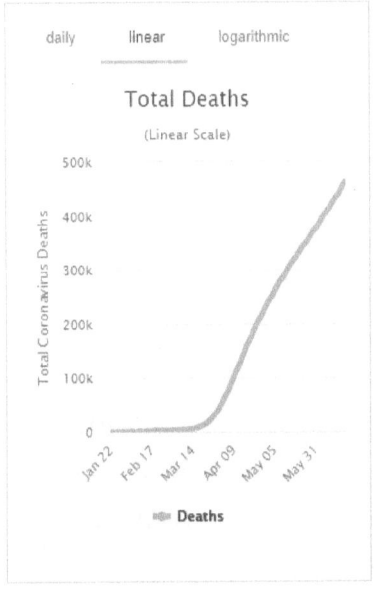

References

[Agrawal et al., 2016] Agrawal AS, Tao X, Algaissi A, et al. Immunization with inactivated Middle East Respiratory Syndrome coronavirus vaccine leads to lung immunopathology on a challenge with live virus. *Hum Vaccin Immunother.* 2016;12(9):2351-2356. doi:10.1080/21645515.2016.1177688

[Chan et al., 2011] Chan KH, Peiris JS, Lam SY, Poon LL, Yuen KY, Seto WH. The effects of temperature and relative humidity on the viability of the SARS coronavirus. Adv Virol **2011**; 2011:734690.

[Chin et al., 2020] Chin AWH, Chu JTS, Perera MRA, et al. Stability of SARS-CoV-2 in different environmental conditions [Letter]. Lancet Microbe **2020**.

[Cohen et al., 1991] Cohen, S., G.M. Williamson, 'Stress and infectious disease in humans,' in: *Psychol. Bull.*, 1991 (109), p. 5-24.

[Dowell SF., 2001] Dowell SF. Seasonal variation in host susceptibility and cycles of certain infectious diseases. *Emerg Infect Dis.* 2001;7(3):369-374. doi:10.3201/eid0703.010301

[Godbout et al., 2006] Godbout JP, Glaser R. Stress-induced immune dysregulation: implications for wound healing, infectious disease and cancer. *J Neuroimmune Pharmacol.* 2006;1(4):421–427.

[He et al., 2015] He D, Chiu AP, Lin Q, Cowling BJ. Differences in the seasonality of Middle East respiratory syndrome coronavirus and influenza in the Middle East. *Int J Infect Dis.* 2015;40:15-16. doi:10.1016/j.ijid.2015.09.012

[Hshieh et al., 2018] Hshieh TT, Inouye SK, Oh ES. Delirium in the Elderly. *Psychiatr Clin North Am.* 2018;41(1):1-17. doi:10.1016/j.psc.2017.10.001

[Kenna et at., 2011] Kenna HA, Poon AW, de los Angeles CP, Koran LM. Psychiatric complications of treatment with corticosteroids: review with case report. *Psychiatry Clin Neurosci.* 2011;65(6):549-560. doi:10.1111/j.1440-1819.2011.02260.x

[Killerby ME et al., 2018] Killerby ME, Biggs HM, Haynes A, et al. Human coronavirus circulation in the United States 2014-2017. *J Clin Virol.* 2018;101:52-56. doi:10.1016/j.jcv.2018.01.019

[Kanzawa et al., 2020] Kanzawa M, Spindler H, Anglemyer A, Rutherford GW. Will Coronavirus Disease 2019 Become Seasonal?. *J Infect Dis.* 2020;222(5):719-721. doi:10.1093/infdis/jiaa345

[Kurlansik et al., 2012] Kurlansik SL, Ibay AD. Seasonal affective disorder. *Am Fam Physician.* 2012;86(11):1037-1041.

[Monto AS et al., 2020] Monto AS, DeJonge P, Callear AP, et al. Coronavirus occurrence and transmission over 8 years in the HIVE cohort of households in Michigan. *J Infect Dis.* 2020;jiaa161. doi:10.1093/infdis/jiaa161

[Nikooie et al., 2019] Nikooie R, Neufeld KJ, Oh ES, et al. Antipsychotics for Treating Delirium in Hospitalized Adults: A Systematic Review. *Ann Intern Med.* 2019;171(7):485-495. doi:10.7326/M19-1860

[O'Hanlon S et al., 2020] O'Hanlon S, Inouye SK. Delirium: a missing piece in the COVID-19 pandemic puzzle [published online ahead of print, 2020 May 6]. *Age Ageing.* 2020;afaa094. doi:10.1093/ageing/afaa094

[Shevlin et al., 2020] Shevlin M, Nolan E, Owczarek M, et al. COVID-19-related anxiety predicts somatic symptoms in the UK population [published online ahead of print, 2020 May 27]. *Br J Health Psychol.* 2020;10.1111/bjhp.12430. doi:10.1111/bjhp.12430

[Sun et al., 2020] Sun Z, Thilakavathy K, Kumar SS, He G, Liu SV. Potential Factors Influencing Repeated SARS Outbreaks in China. *Int J Environ Res Public Health.* 2020;17(5):1633. Published 2020 Mar 3. doi:10.3390/ijerph17051633

[Tseng et al., 2012] Tseng CT, Sbrana E, Iwata-Yoshikawa N, et al. Immunization with SARS coronavirus vaccines leads to pulmonary immunopathology on challenge with the SARS virus [published correction appears in PLoS One. 2012;7(8). doi:10.1371/annotation/2965cfae-b77d-4014-8b7b-236e01a35492]. *PLoS One.* 2012;7(4):e35421. doi:10.1371/journal.pone.0035421 [van Doremalen et al., 2020] van Doremalen N, Bushmaker T, Morris DH, et al. Aerosol and surface stability of SARS-CoV-2 as compared with SARS-CoV-1. N Engl J Med **2020**; 382:1564–7.

[Yang et al., 2002] Yang EV, Glaser R. Stress-associated immunomodulation and its implications for responses to vaccination. Expert Rev Vaccines. 2002;1(4):453-459. doi:10.1586/14760584.1.4.453

[Zimmermann et al., 2019] Zimmermann P, Curtis N. Factors That Influence the Immune Response to Vaccination. *Clin Microbiol Rev.* 2019;32(2):e00084-18. Published 2019 Mar 13. doi:10.1128/CMR.00084-18

12. Where oh Where is the Virus in Europe?

June 23, 2020

	Today	Total
Cases worldwide	138.975	9.189.875
Deaths worldwide	3.880	473.484

Summer is dawning. The sun knows it all over Europe, as do the people who seem to live in a full post-corona era. So do many individuals in the US. What can we expect?

Did the virus come and go?

Are Europeans and US citizens awakening from a one-stand nightmare? Are we safe to get on with our work, life, unprotected mass gatherings, and partying on the streets from now on and for a very long time? Experts say 'no.' Many people don't care. Others are super-anxious.

So, is it all behind us? Of course not.

Worldwide acceleration

With 303 deaths in Europe and 363 in the US yesterday, things have indeed been much worse just two months ago. At the same time, over the last month and continuing, there is a gradual speeding up in the numbers of daily cases and deaths worldwide. The virus hasn't left humanity.

With a low herd immunity everywhere (+/- 5-10%), the virus still has much leeway.

Invisible = inexistent?

So it seems to many. It makes me think of another invisibility, that of nonconscious subconceptual processing. 'Subconceptual' because it's about mental patterns that can hardly or not be caught in well-delineated concepts. Scientifically, it is how the brain works. It's there. It's our +/- 80 billion neurons firing and patterning away all the time, even while sleeping. Neurocognitive scientists speak of a 'universe inside.' We continuously see through it, but we don't see it. Yet. It is factual. It is how the brain – thus also the mind – influences the way you breathe, how your heart pounds, and when you feel tired or energetic.

And indeed, there is also a large scientifically known impact on the immune system. This way, we come close to how the body reacts to the virus.

Invisible, but not nonexistent at all.

Seasonal corona

One scenario is that this coronavirus behaves like all other known coronaviruses: seasonally. In Europe and the US, this means a peak in wintertime, an almost disappearance in the summertime. This pattern reenacts itself as it is year after year.

An exception that proves the rule recently happened in a slaughterhouse in northwestern Germany, with an outbreak of more than 1000 cases, a 6th of the personnel. In many slaughterhouses, people work in stressful circumstances in an artificial winter climate. Not surprisingly, such factories in the US show the same pattern, including proneness to COVID-19.

Even outside of slaughterhouses, of course, we see individual COVID-cases. So, is a second wave possible during the summer? I would say yes. Is it probable? I would say no. In any case, much less probable than in wintertime. If there is an upsurge during the summer, we should be extremely wary about what's to come. It spells disaster.

Surprisingly, little is known about the precise mechanism for seasonal fluctuations. Influencing factors are social behavior, temperature, and probably the amount of sunlight.

Another factor is how our brain/mind reacts to this.

Here we go again. Invisible, not inexistent. Yet psychology may also explain why the drop in corona casualties is so surprisingly dramatic right now, right here. We come from a whirlpool – individual and social – in which the virus was present as well as our universe inside. [See chapter 'COVID whirlpool' in *Minding Corona*]

> Placebo: a dummy pill acts positively even though there is no active substance inside. According to scientists, there is more placebo than pharmacology in many present-day Western medications. The power of true placebo resides in expectations, deeper meaning, and other mind-related factors.

> Nocebo: quite the same but with negative action. Nocebo can be part of a whirlpool that drags people unnecessarily down.

Of course, this doesn't mean there is no pharmacology nor virus. What it does mean is scary.

We may get into the same whirlpool, even worse.

Time will tell. There is no scientific experimental proof, but many factors point to this direction. There is no doubt about the substantial influence of the mind on the progression of viral diseases, including AIDS, as is shown by much academic research. There is also no doubt about the substantial influence of the mind on the immune system in many ways. See my book *Your Mind as Cure* for a broad explanation.

As to COVID-19, as rapidly as we have evolved from disaster to blue sky, equally rapidly we may get into disaster mode again. Our mind helps in both ways.

So, what will happen?

Looking into a crystal ball, I only see crystal. Peering into the future, I see a very bleak landscape with panic, loss of control, and a new lockdown in Europe and the US.

The carefree attitude of many people now may heighten this. It brings a direct danger in pockets of infection. It also keeps the virus present or might make it even more widespread. Note that the virus was present in European drinking water already in December before anyone got ill.

At this very moment, it may be spreading in many places. Invisibly. In the corona season, starting from October and (depending on the type) peaking around February, it may surge from many places simultaneously. Then, what about contact tracing?

And what about vaccination?

A vaccine developed in time would be miraculous but not a miracle. Take Influenza, for example, for which the vaccination doesn't give full protection but only a bit less than half.

Also, the natural immunity after corona infection lasts six to twelve months. Herd immunity may be short-lived. More bleakness: What if a new wave comes with a viral mutation into a deadlier strain, as happened with the Spanish flu a century ago?

Back to summertime

Let's enjoy it, but let's not waste our time. Surely, the pharmaceutical industry is looking for more useful medication. Let's hope for that. My take is the psychological one. I have published a book about this, *Minding Corona*, to be found on Amazon for $3 as an e-book. Also, I have developed an app to be used as mental support, free to everyone, to be found on https://aurelis.org/aurelis-app. It will also be available soon in Google and Apple stores.

In my view, the one and the other together will save many lives. This will make me a happy man, although also a sad one for future-peering so much.

If you want to help, please read the book, download the app, and reach out. There is a lot to be done for our own sake soon, for the world right away, day after day. Also, experiences elsewhere in this regard may help us when needed.

We are not out of the woods.

13. Winter of COVID

June 25, 2020

	Today	Total
Cases worldwide	172.383	9.566.124
Deaths worldwide	5.071	485.704

Second Wave Corona? One big or several smaller ones? While we don't know what is to happen, we can search for arguments.

Quoting Andrea Ammon

Director of the European Centre for Disease Prevention and Control, 21 May 2020:

> "It's not a question of if there will be a renewed surge but when and how big."

That means hoping for the best but preparing for the worst. The latter is a likely resurgence of COVID-19, across countries, through regions, in towns and communities. Including the renewed choice between lockdowns and lives.

Much depends on caution.

But how to be cautious and what works in caution, again, we don't know.

For instance, statistics clearly show that lockdown works. There is no doubt. It may have saved and is still saving millions of lives worldwide. It was/is a good thing!

But statistics don't tell us precisely how it works. The biggest issue that I see – as to the central theme in *Minding Corona* – is whether it works conceptually or subconceptually. Both, indeed, which makes it a question of proportionality.

Subconceptual?

To repeat in a few words: 'subconceptual' points to mental patterns that hardly or not need to reach conscious awareness in order to have meaningful effects upon mind and body. Like something may be bothering you and you aren't consciously aware of it, yet you can feel a resulting tension or pain somewhere in your body. This is scientifically uncontroversial in many fields of chronic pain and more. [see *Your Mind as Cure*]

Lockdown may subconceptually work by giving people the confidence that things will be all right. This confidence provides a message in the way of a placebo. It can have a positive effect if deeply felt. It may keep one out of a mind-body whirlpool.

> [Whirlpool image: ten meters from it, it's innocuous. Go ten meters further from it, and you're entirely out of danger. Get the same distance towards it, and it drags you down. Yet ten meters from it, if you don't see it, this may be hard to fathom.]

I won't explain nocebo again. It may also play a substantial role in what is happening in COVID-19 in the recent past and near future, in reverse to the previous. It may push people deeper into the whirlpool.

In this way, we are talking Winter of COVID. Since the world cannot go in lockdown again and again, we will need to face the virus head-on with little herd-immunity.

As to the Minding Corona premise, if not taken into account, this would be a second whirlpool.

The first wave happened surprisingly abrupt in several parts of the world. At least in Western Europe, at the moment of writing, it has also subsided surprisingly suddenly.

Just looking at this, it's imaginable that a second wave will surge surprisingly abrupt.

'Surprisingly' means that we don't know precisely all the relevant parameters. Those deemed important may play a secondary role. On the other hand, an interplay of factors may give rise to a self-enhancing pattern, described by me as a whirlpool of mind and body elements.

As I show in many domains, mind and body naturally go together in one structure, namely a human being as a complex living organism. Not a mechanism; an organism in which complexity and emergence play substantial roles. The COVID-19 whirlpool appears within this structure. Take each of the elements on its own, and the whirlpool doesn't emerge. The whole is way much more than the sum of the parts. This may be the case for a surprising amount of other disorders as well.

Invisible mind in an invisible whirlpool

In the COVID-19 story until now, I haven't seen the mind described as a causal element. There has not been any clarification of this as one can do from cutting-edge neurocognitive science, and as I have done so myself in the first part of *The Journey Towards Compassionate A.I.*

So, logically, there has not been any description of the whirlpool in which the virus and the mind can play a determining role in several respects. Therefore, there has not been any description from this insight into what happened and may happen again. And, indeed, what is happening in different parts of the world right now.

Why can next winter in Europe be the worst?

In a previous text, I mentioned the seasonal curves of other coronaviruses as they have been academically investigated. These show a sharp seasonality, peaking in the winter, with maxima in January and February. In the springtime of 2020, COVID-19 has taken Europe by storm mainly from mid-march. Even a bit later in the US. If the present coronavirus acts the same as these other ones, we may have witnessed only the tail of the beast. Over the year from now on, we may see the whole beast, with its belly at the start of 2021.

Also, the new coronavirus came after the Influenza season. Next time, both will come in combination. This does not mean that two half-diseases will make one person having a disease. It involves two diseases at the same time. For the immune system: two enemies to battle at the same time. Let's hope this description is exaggerated. If not, then the cohort of vulnerable people will be bigger; the ages of the severely diseased will be younger; complications and deaths more frequent.

Also, there will be, as every year, a lot of common colds in all age groups. An instance of common cold may be from another virus. Still, the sneezing and the coughing are there. Combine this with the fact – as researchers agree [Nature, May 2020] – that children have viral loads comparable to those of grown-ups, only don't get COVID themselves [BI et al., 2020], they will be sneezing and coughing the coronaviruses around in the autumn and winter, more than in the previous springtime. Put them in schools together, and you have one big time bomb. Other respiratory viruses are known to circulate in schools and daycare centers. To the kids themselves, this may be mainly one more but not to their (grand)parents.

Dear God, let me be wrong.

Also, with much common cold around, it will be more difficult to ask people to self-isolate when symptoms appear. The first symptoms of common cold and COVID-19 are pretty much the same. Note again that a person is most infectious during the few days before and after the appearance of symptoms. A gigantic amount of testing might relieve this, but it has its specific problems.

Also, in what happens in the US now (huge and rising numbers of cases and deaths), one may see mainly the power of the whirlpool without full force of the virus which also there is to come in a few months.

Also, all the previous together may make people believe that it's all out of control. One can see the whirlpool turning.

Also, economists warn that the economy cannot take a second lockdown in the way of the first. It will be a different story. Businesses are barely surviving now. Money cannot be artificially made by governments ad infinitum. So, will we again wait too long and need to lockdown anyway with tremendous health costs on top?

Has the virus already become milder?

As a glimmer of hope, according to some researchers, COVID-19 (the disorder) seems to have become milder in the few months from the start of the first wave in Europe. This needs confirmation. Some conclude from this that the virus itself has changed already so that a second wave would be less severe, and we shouldn't worry too much.

The latter is true. We shouldn't worry too much, for the anxiety adds to the whirlpool's energy. In this sense, warning for a huge second wave may even be self-fulfilling. I hope this text is not a part of that. In my view, openness and inner strength are also preferable in this respect.

But one cannot conclude any evolution of the virus itself from the evolution of the disorder. Anyway, the most significant part of the disorder is not related to the virus but the immune response. So, this seems to have become milder. That is foreseeable from the *Minding Corona* premise. People gradually get used to disasters, even to big ones, with time. Such is also seen in wartime.

Besides, could the virus itself in its replication thrift learn so quickly, and adapt to the fact that killing its host hampers its own replication? Here too, it's relevant to point out that the over-reaction of the host frequently occurs when the viral load itself has already diminished. It would be surprising that the virus learns from a projection into the future.

A diminishing strength of the disease would be one more indication that the mind indeed influences the immune over-reaction against the virus.

In second-wave, this may be crucial. One may try to relieve the relevant factor. 'Anxiety' is a broad term for this, too broad in my view, but still a good direction to start with. It's also a multifaceted term. We can use it further on [see also: "Motivation Without Anxiety"] to expound upon how to tackle a second wave or any wave.

After a vacation from the virus, at the strike of the second wave, people may again start from a full-panic mode. Will it be less or more than the first time? Much of this is up to our thinking about it and our taking action without delay.

The concept of 'negative carrier'

Can a person be a carrier of the virus for a long time, be infectious, and yet all this time test negative? Or can a virus go under the testing radar for a while to then reappear and provoke an infection from inside out?

There are a lot of 'ifs' in this. With a new virus, anything is possible, but not anything is probable. Let's think about it.

According to an article in the British Medical Journal [BMJ, May 2020], a "systematic review of the accuracy of COVID-19 tests reported false-negative rates of between 2% and 29%, based on negative RT-PCR tests which were positive on repeat testing." This is quite high. However, as a Gold standard, repeat testing is bound to underestimate the real rate of false negatives, possibly to a considerable degree. Indeed, how would one rule out a 'negative carrier'? If the test is its own Gold standard, a negative carrier will remain a negative carrier until, of course, he becomes a positive carrier. This way, we cannot rule out the existence of negative carriers.

So, yes, they may exist in principle. We don't know how long they can remain so, let alone do we know if or when they can be or become contagious.

What surely does exist is asymptomatic transmission. Studies already documented this in March. It has been pointed out as a reason why the virus has been hard to control. It is a reason why someone should stay at home when someone else in the household may have coronavirus infection. Research among staff in the hospitals run by a leading NHS trust in the north of England found that 7% had coronavirus on testing but had no symptoms and thus posed a risk to patients. According to NHS bosses, "Up to a fifth of patients with COVID-19 in several hospitals contracted the disease while being treated there for another illness." [The Guardian, May 2020].

How many more were/are negative carriers? We don't know.

The enigma Africa

Of course, the virus is very much present in Africa. In a country like Nigeria, for instance, with relatively few COVID cases, not one province is exempt. How to explain the difference between Africans-in-Africa and African Americans (as well as those in Brazil), where cases are soaring disproportionately more in black communities than white?

Is one factor the exposure to racism and its implications (additional daily stress, job opportunities, poor neighborhoods, incarceration)? Are Africans-in-Africa less prone to succumb to the stress-virus due to a different relationship to stress? They may be equally yet differently stressed. Stress is a multifaceted phenomenon. I agree: this way, everything and nothing can be explained. That doesn't make it less crucial to try to find a rational path in the stressional landscape.

Is it because of a stricter and earlier lockdown? African countries have much experience with other infectious diseases in this respect. But how long can they stay in lockdown economy-wise? Opening up and with the virus already being present all over Africa, will they also see a whirlpool ravaging the continent? In the Minding Corona premise, we should be prepared. Once getting out of control, the whirlpool emerges.

The same may be the case in Eastern Europe: stricter and earlier lockdown, imposed on people who probably adhere to rules more swiftly than many Western Europeans and US citizens. More fear perhaps and less anxiety, which makes a crucial difference towards the individual and social whirlpool phenomena. But can the economy survive a repeated lockdown? Being massively confronted with the virus and minimal herd immunity, will people be immune?

Very upsetting!

It means that with eyes closed, we are heading to a possible yet preventable disaster. And, indeed, different parts of the world are there right now.

Costing many economic assets. For many businesses, a financial knockout.

Costing many lives, directly and indirectly COVID-related.

Costing many survivors' longtime health problems.

These are challenging times.

References

[BI et al., 2020] Bi, Q. *et al. Lancet Infect. Dis.* https://doi.org/10.1016/S1473-3099(20)30287-5 (2020).

[BMJ, May 2020] www.bmj.com/content/369/bmj.m1808.

[Nature, May 2020] www.nature.com/articles/d41586-020-01354-0#ref-CR1.

[The Guardian, May 2020] www.theguardian.com/world/2020/may/17/hospital-patients-england-coronavirus-covid-19.

14. Motivation Without Anxiety in Corona Times

June 27, 2020

	Today	Total
Cases worldwide	**176.568**	**10.075.115**
Deaths worldwide	**4.891**	**500.624**

[There are a few links in this text towards other blog posts by me. You can either click through or go to https://aurelis.org/blog and search on the exact string.]

Motivation may be the single most crucial factor in the whole COVID story. Yet it doesn't get the attention it deserves.

General motivation principles

Corona times form a good occasion to learn about what is more generally applicable. Also, such times may show us the importance of striving for correctness in these principles. Many lives are directly concerned. One shouldn't be coy about this.

Every motivational mistake costs human lives and health.

Motivation drives us.

It does so in significant issues as well as in the smallest one.

Without motivation, there is no motion, no change, no action. Anything you do comes from your motivation to do so and not otherwise. If you read this, you are motivated to read. If you keep reading, you are even more motivated to read this. Your motivation keeps you reading.

Otherwise, you would have stopped reading at the previous sentence.

Nonconscious

Motivation can be conscious or nonconscious, or so it seems. But it's not true. Motivation is always nonconscious. 'Motivation' in consciousness is as much a product of the underlying motivation as any other action being the result of where it comes from.

Otherwise, you could force yourself to be motivated. It would be a conscious decision to get motivated. And it isn't. You can try it out at any time, taking something for which you are not motivated. Then try to force yourself into motivation just by the blank thought. Snap your finger and be motivated. Snap it again and be motivated for the reverse. And again.

You see, it doesn't work that way.

The same is valid for motivating others.

It also doesn't work that way. Meaning: you cannot force another person to be motivated. You can only force him to do something. But that's not motivation. It's coercion — big difference.

If you start working from the idea of active motivation, you cannot motivate anyone, ever. In the other case, a motivational universe opens itself.

And now we have entered a corona era, in which motivation is of utmost importance mainly for two reasons:

- to let people keep social distance
- to keep vulnerable people more distant from the whirlpool phenomenon

These may seem not deeply related, but as we will see, in depth, the same principles are crucial.

Superficial characteristics of motivation are not relevant.

For instance, one can try to 'speak the language' of the person-to-be-motivated. But if it's not from the heart, it also feels this way. Even more, it may feel like manipulation, which it is. [see: "Difference between Motivation and Manipulation"] This diminishes trust and creates anxiety. That's precisely what we should avoid, as it's energy for the negative whirlpool.

But 'speaking the language' can, of course, also be done from the heart. In this case, the language is an opening towards the heart. It's there that the chemistry works, in 'deep to deep communication,' from heart to heart. Such communication motivates, even if at the superficial level, people may intellectually disagree.

The conclusion is that 'speaking the language' is not relevant as a superficial characteristic. Important is how you speak and crucial in this again is depth.

So, should one 'speak the language' to be motivational? Yes and no. Since a lot of speaking and writing about it is merely superficial, it detracts from what's important. This includes every study that doesn't reach depth in the domain of motivation. No wonder there is so much contradiction and short-lived theorizing about motivation and, among other things, motivational leadership. [see: "Motivational Team-Leading?"]

"We're in this together."

Are we? Yes, but with differences. One can see this regional or worldwide. Of course, there are immense differences in healthcare provisions. These are important now and will become even more so shortly. We are all in this together. If the virus is kept at bay in Europe but, let's say, becomes rampantly prevalent in Africa, then Europe will not one moment be safe either.

Seeing that we're all in the same big boat is not just a question of altruism. Together, we are sailing through space on our little blue planet. We are more and more bound to be together, and that's a good thing!

Togetherness plays to the feeling of empathy. Some may feel this more readily for people in their direct environment; others readily feel empathy much more broadly. The extremes of this continuum may mistrust each other, thinking that the other side of the continuum – becoming a duality this way – has no empathy and, thus, in times of corona, will worsen the situation. For instance, one can see this in the issue of 'health versus economy.' In reality, health and economy go together. It would be motivating for all to keep hammering on this. There is no modern healthcare without economy. There is no modern economy without healthy people.

Pre-existing divisions – which always start with inner division – may heighten through this misconception. This makes it even more necessary to enhance the togetherness in corona times, not the division. If some good can come out of it all, it's from the experience of being in this together.

Social distancing drives people physically apart from each other. This can be balanced with social togetherness, the feeling of being in this together. I hope that in due time, the social distancing may disappear, while the social togetherness remains.

Deeper values motivate.

At the same time, deeper values unite. We all want health. We all naturally – unless as the result of some deep frustration – want to care for ourselves and others. We all want a world without a pandemic. Even more, we all want to be deeply happy, and that is only possible if others are happy.

Having secured one's deeper values heightens deep happiness. Deep happiness heightens inner strength, which strengthens the immune system. I say this with confidence, not from specific experimental research but from many indications that themselves are scientifically validated.

The opposite is inner dissociation [see: "Inner Dissociation is NEVER OK!"]. For instance, a smoker may want to quit smoking, but internally, he doesn't want to – precisely because of his addiction. So, there's an inner divide, a fight against oneself, provoking stress. The smoker feels it and relieves it by smoking, and so on. The same mechanism is at play with many other issues. The result is a chronically stressed individual. Put age or another risk on top, and you get an individual prone to succumbing to a virus that has found stressed organisms as its niche. The present coronavirus may be the most advanced in this until now.

Motivating people in corona-era also has as a valid goal the diminishment of this inner divide and stress. In the long term and...

in the short term. How-to?

I cannot be consistent without referring to the free Aurelis app, of course, available at https://aurelis.org/aurelis-app. I had this in mind when developing the app in the first place. If one would analyze the ten immersive exercises (five 'mild' and five 'severe'), one would see that they are not mere relaxations. They are oriented explicitly toward supporting people in finding their inner strength within stressful circumstances. There is no time to turn around the bush. It's hands-on support, with stress and challenge already present. One can do the exercises and redo them while listening to them or just thinking about them. The goal is what comes out of you, not what you put into yourself through listening to me. It's your inner strength, your mental landscape. Roaming there, you find the motivation to live and be healthy, and on top of that, to live a healthy life. Is this asking too much?

The app can work directly. It can also work by sheer knowledge that it's available as support in times of trouble. I would recommend having it available indeed, doing exercises at least a bit in time, so that you know what to expect. Also, it's like art or at least a handcraft/mind-craft. By exercising, one learns to use the app more efficiently and with better result. This way, when needed, you can skip the learning curve. It's there. It's ready for you. And as said, it's freely available.

Beside the app, in the short term, I think motivation starts with avoiding de-motivation. Any physician learns to 'primum non nocere.' First of all, do not harm. We can read it here as: "Do not de-motivate if you can avoid such." For instance, one can try to make people wear face masks by saying that "You will be guilty if you don't wear one and we will all pay the price for your misconduct." This boggles my mind. Its political correctness is not relevant. It creates much resistance and, sooner or later, precisely what one tries to avoid, for sure.

The virus is still among us. If we don't take care, many more people will get sick and die. We are sure of that. One may try to make people consume more by neglecting or hiding this. Simultaneously cajoling them into wearing face masks 'for the purpose of health' is transparently inconsistent and provokes much anxiety. See: now next to each other are living those very anxious and those very careless or even hostile, and a division that nobody wants.

So, how to make people wear face masks?

By being open as much as possible. Even better but much more difficult, by being Open. [see: "The Future is Open"

Being open is trying to get messages out that are acceptable to everyone. These are mainly positive ones. Not "You are guilty and should be punished" but, for instance, "You are a responsible person and deserve admiration if you indeed take responsibility for the sake of others, including your (grand)parents and those of your neighbors."

And the economy? Surely, wearing face masks now will enable us to avoid or postpone the next lockdown. Wearing face masks is an element in our collective battle to save our economy. There is no contradiction with health.

In my experience, openness to depth almost always comes together with an openness to a level where one can say 'yes' to anything that passes by. No this-versus-that. No zero-sum based polity in many issues. Different people want the same things in very different ways. Still, these are the same things and we can say 'yes' to each other without neglecting oneself or anyone else.

In times of corona, this not only saves lives. It also saves the economy of today and tomorrow. There are lessons to be learned for the future.

See also the appendix '20 reasons to wear your face mask.'

Japan, intriguingly

Japan = big crowded cities (37 million in Tokyo) with notoriously packed transportation lines, no enforced lockdown, little testing (0.27% of the population), more elderly per capita than anywhere in the world, fair shares of disease. Japan has many characteristics for an outbreak of the disaster, yet it has almost none of it. Antibody testing shows that only 0.1-0.25% of the population has been infected. How come?

It's intriguing. Instead of an enforced lockdown, Japanese people were asked, on a voluntary basis, to avoid the 'three Cs': enclosed spaces, crowded places, and close contacts. And they voluntarily complied, not surprisingly. As a people, the Japanese are known to be caring for the collective. They don't need anxiety-provoking messages. As a second consequence, they're also not generally anxious that others will not care. They know that others will voluntarily comply. They're in the challenge together.

Is this morally better or worse? That's the most challenging question that I will not answer. But in times of COVID, it may have a double positive consequence: 1) People do social-distancing at every level, and 2) The whirlpool gets fueled much less by nocebo expectations, anxiety, and COVID-related stress. On the contrary, knowing that there is a massive collective effort for the good of all may actively diminish the whirlpool's energy.

In search of a 'factor X' (or so-called 'mindo') that would prove the people's superiority over others, well, I acknowledge that the deeper mind can indeed be brought in relation to this. There's a lesson to be learned for all of us, being the others. But also for the Japanese themselves, I guess. A feeling of exceptionality may lead to negative as well as positive results. A sense of superiority is already on the verge of the negative. With bad leadership, this makes one prone to manipulation. In the near future, it might make the Japanese over-confident in their apparent COVID-immunity, with much negative energy coming from this loss of confidence.

So, does the Japanese situation align with the premise of this book? It is not a proof, but intriguingly consistent. Taking a look at the image in the appendix 'The COVID-Whirlpool-Drawing,' one can see two main sides: the conceptual more at the left, the subconceptual more at the right. The Japanese have stress all right, but probably much less COVID-related. Stress is not a simple thing. On the contrary, it's very complex and multidimensional.

We see in the example of Japan how a whirlpool without fuel from either side stays astonishingly tiny. In principle, this is possible everywhere. So, what can make the difference between a giant whirlpool and a tiny one?

Motivation without anxiety

Striving towards such has two positive sides:

- This amounts to relieving anxiety.
- This forces one to get into deep motivation-mode, by not thinking that 'anxiety will keep the people within law and order so I don't have to do my job as a leader.'

For this, real motivation needs to be achieved. It's a long-term endeavor. Some of it can be put into practice right away. The long and short term should not be intermingled. They have the same underlying principles but a different concrete way of accomplishment. One shouldn't ask in the short term what is only possible in the long term.

Inner dissociation creates anxiety, different from fear. [see: "Difference between Fear and Anxiety"] Anxiety is probably the biggest source of stress – or is it eventually the same thing? Also stress at work, 'boss stress' (not of the boss himself so much, but of those who get bossed around) is anxiety-related. It goes deeper than just having fear for the pain when the boss will hit you – which bosses generally don't do anymore. But making people anxious? Sure they do. It's a frequently used instrument by bosses to get things done.

Contrary to this, motivation without anxiety is an instrument of leadership. Can we derive from this that leadership is of utmost importance in corona times?

Yes we can.

Open Leadership saves many lives.

See *Open Leadership – Read&*Do for more ideas about this.

Does this coincide with present-day experience?

15. Mind the Denial

June 30, 2020

	Today	Total
Cases worldwide	174.264	10.577.756
Deaths worldwide	5.072	513.186

More and more, I wonder why it is so very, very hard for many to see the mind in what is happening with corona worldwide.

Why?

In view of the possible collapse of the world economy and devastation of the health of millions, we should cherish every straw of possible relief. Conceptually, we do so. Subconceptually, I see nothing of the sort. It fills me with desperation.

On top of this, for short-sighted economic reasons, the world is presently taking risks into the unknown, risks that may backfire immensely. In writing previous texts, I have made it clear, to myself at least, that we are dancing at the brink of the real precipice that we haven't seen yet. Economy-wise, many countries cannot take a second hit, including prosperous ones like China, the US, and European countries. In the second, larger hit, a renewed general lockdown will be necessary and impossible.

In all this mayhem, it is understandable that one wants this nightmare to go away, but one cannot just wish it away. Europe and the US seem full of people who, one way or another, think they can. Acting as if the virus is away doesn't make it go away. A child knows that, from around an age of four. So, why don't we <u>collectively</u> see this quite obvious precipice? Why didn't we see the one we just fell into — even while many are still falling? And why don't we see the mind in this?

Attentive readers of *Minding Corona* may, by now, already give me some reasons. Indeed, it is hard to see the mind in anything. Can a seer see himself if he doesn't have access to a proper mirror? Also, we encountered body-mind dualism and the denial of nonconscious yet meaningful mental processing. Our blindfolds to these factors are culturally and profoundly embedded, thus with many associations into many domains. While at the surface, these domains seem independent, they are, in reality, very interdependent. This is also how we treat the world. It is also how we treat ourselves, for instance, in healthcare: as a mechanism of separate sub-elements: a heart, a brain, an immune system, even 'a mind.' At many levels, the reality is much more interdependent than what many people hold on to.

Denial?

A lot has been written about denial, also in a social context. Denial by fear of having to change one's usual ways of doing and relating, by blindness, incapacity, or unwillingness to see or even look whether there is anything to see in the first place. Denial by an act of faith: technology will solve our problems, so we don't have to delve into anything that might turn out to be a cesspit (thus, the cesspit remains). And didn't it work out well (denying the cesspit) in the past? Denial by fear of losing one's status, money, reputation, and carrier, of losing the prospect of a future that one has imagined already so vividly — better keep the dream a while longer. Denial by habit of denial.

Denial because it's hard work to change an existing paradigm. Indeed, even nature wants it so because it's costly to change paradigm. Nature is a tinkerer; evolution changes in little steps, trying to live life in the moment. A big change can be too costly and mean the end of everything – not sustainable, of course.

Being part of nature, we naturally tend to be in denial of many things as long as – in our perception – the cost of the alternative is higher than the cost of staying put. No revolution today, please. One can see this in science as anywhere else. Notably, Thomas Kuhn has written about the difficulty of scientific paradigm shifts.

Additionally disconcerting is the issue that denial may be a genuine part of the whirlpool. I mean with this not just a neglecting of the facts, but a plain not-willing-to-see. The risk may be too disconcerting to face, or the message too ego-engulfing. As a matter of fact, this is extremely dangerous in the present situation. Sadly, it is not a future danger that we can still totally avoid. It is ongoing.

Following nature

Yet if nature wants it so, then – in the long term – I think we should follow that. Is this surprising? Of course, this doesn't mean we should keep ourselves in denial and let the virus wreak havoc. The cost of the latter is way too high. Fortunately, following nature and having it our way may go together. At least, if we succeed in getting past any straightforward denial of our true selves – nature within us – that is getting increasingly and immensely costly. We are organisms, not mechanisms. Neither should we treat workers as mechanisms. We shouldn't treat our personal health as that of a mechanism. We should also not treat animals as mechanisms. It is unnatural. We try to impose a mechanical paradigm upon nature. Nature resists. We feel it in an ever-increasing number of burnouts. We see it in climate change. We encounter it in this viral pandemic and more to come. It will not stop until we learn.

The present conundrum (not only COVID, but also the broader context) may even be seen as a test from nature. If we – as a human species – pass this test, we can get propelled into a bright future. If we don't, we'll have to redo the academic year and try better. Of course, nature is not a professor. It doesn't even think as we do. But it made us, didn't it? So, there is something one could very broadly call 'intelligence,' one way or another. I use 'test' metaphorically. Still, we might not pass it.

Underlying principle: us

At the basis of the COVID-19-crisis lies the same as what risks making it much worse, as well as why it is hard for many to see the mind in this, even while it's increasingly obvious if one cares to keenly look.

One may wonder why it's so hard to get beyond the denial of one's own deeper mind. The world is on fire, and we have to look the dragon into the eyes. I did that, and I saw a princess. I'm talking about nonconscious, subconceptual mental processing itself, the 'thing inside that is invisible.' And I'm not surprised by this since I earned a Ph.D. in medical science on this subject. It drives us in mind and body. If we don't see that it is who we are, then it seems like a stranger driving us. Denying that, the stranger may become a symbolic dragon. Since one cannot see a symbol (I mean, what is symbolized), the situation may become precarious. We then 'see' the dragon in something outside, whether it's a virus or a person from another culture, religion or race. Of course, those things or people are really there. The problem starts when they become recipients of negative symbolism.

It's frightening and so near, and so frightening because it's near. At the same time, through denial and resistance, it's also functionally far away. Then it's terrifying because it's far away and unknown and strange *and*, at the same time, still so near. Nothing can be nearer.

This is what we collectively need to see in order to pass the exam with distinction. The immediate reward: much less suffering shortly. A long-term bonus: getting to know ourselves better and see how our self-ignorance is bringing us this and many other problems. Many of these are also health-related.

How is it possible?

How can the influence of the mind on the body be so significant? And how can it be so invisible to almost everybody, even while we are witnessing the immensely dire result? These seem two different questions, each mind-boggling on its own. Each of both seems very weird. The combination, therefore, even stranger.

I see behind both the same principle that I call 'inner dissociation' and the tension that this provokes. In short, we are still organisms, but we tend to manage ourselves as if we were mechanisms. With more technology, we could handle ourselves better as who we are, but we do the reverse.

Thus, our technology is a double-edged sword. One can see this in health-related technology and broader.

Natural evolution has engendered consciousness. The human being stands at the pinnacle of consciousness. Culture and technology have propelled us even further in the direction of conscious, conceptual thinking. Super, but meanwhile, we are a body-mind that, for the most part, does *not* work conceptually. The fact that we don't properly see this and don't live accordingly creates a tremendous tension. So, it's not just the case that there is a huge tension *and* we don't see where it comes from and is going to. The tension is present *precisely because* we don't see it.

In history-in-a-nutshell, there have been more promising times in this regard. In the 18th century, one can think of the first phase of Western Enlightenment, which has been engulfed by the ensuing, more conceptual phase. Nearing the end of the 19th century, one can think of a growing interest in suggestion and 'the nonconscious,' which has been hijacked by the more conceptual Freudian psychoanalysis. In the 20th century, I think of 'the sixties' as a movement that has evaporated into the background. There were opportunities. There still are. If such opportunities are not taken, we get disasters. In my view, the present shows us a consequence of mainly this. For suitable relief, we need to have insight, not only as an intellectual endeavor but as what by itself amounts to the diminishment of the inner dissociation. In the seeing lies the relieving. In doctor's parlance: the diagnosis is the therapy. As to now, we don't diagnose, and we don't cure. In my view, the present shows us a consequence of mainly this.

We direly need to get to know who we are.

Active denial

'Active' is meant here in the sense that a person may consciously, half-consciously, or nonconsciously distance himself from an insight or a necessary action. The ethical conscience of that same person would not go into denial, but the person knows or feels or intuits that his giving-into would lead to the need for unwanted choices. Thus, he doesn't merely deny. He also takes action (or an actively doing-nothing, an active not-thinking) not to see 'the truth,' especially when seeing part of it would lead to an obvious need for more action, insight, and change. Even more so when a substantial portion of what is being denied is deeply related to the meaning-level, most of all one's professional or personal status.

> *[I put 'the truth' in quotation marks. There is no room for a philosophical discussion. In short, this is mainly about a direction, an intention.]*

This may eventually act like a kind of little whirlpool within the person-in-denial who is no longer in full control. An astonishing amount of energy may be needed to draw that person out of it. In many cases, it's even better not to waste energy and to look, instead, for people who are not in active denial. Even more, a person in active denial may become loudly aggressive when brought into head-on contact with what he is denying.

Yet more 'energetic' is an active collective denial. If nobody talks about something, then it's not present in a functional way. Being functionally absent, of course, nobody talks about it, which makes it even harder to be seen. The result is that one doesn't see it because one doesn't see it. The experience happened to me when delving for a while in the scientific virology literature, in which – as far as I delved – the mind was so absent that I caught myself thinking in a mind-absent way. It's contagious.

Whirlpools like this are mainly subconceptual phenomena. Their management needs an approach that is different from a rational-conceptual one. Crucial in this is not to drop rationality, but to enhance it by taking into account subconceptual mental processing as well. The result is a considerable step towards reality. Also, one may progress towards science that better explores this reality. In medical science – among others – the rewards will be immense, but the necessary changes will be essential.

Looking at history, much active denial is to be foreseen when writing it.

So, who listens?

Maybe you, dear reader, are listening while reading. Then please try to comprehend it as well as possible. Don't take anything at face value.

Also, please help to get this message out.

Second-wave whirlpool

I hope that the whirlpool image lets many people see more easily that behind the first wave, there's a second one approaching and which may be even (much) larger. Due to the whirlpool-phenomenon and a large part of this being our invisible deeper mind and inner dissociation, the second wave may be invisible until it's astonishingly near. We had this experience just a few months ago. My impression in Europe at this moment is one of active collective denial. The same may be relevant in the US.

A COVID second wave will probably be delineated after the facts. Until then, it's challenging to distinguish between pockets of the first wave and a full-blown second or even third wave. To me, 'second' denotes an upsurge after a period in which most people live in a happy atmosphere of thinking that the beast has gone, and only its tail is felt. This atmosphere marks the difference and can also play a substantial role in engendering the new wave. Look at it this way: the whirlpool turns slowly and gets neglected until, from inside out, it has amassed much energy anew. When it starts visibly turning again, it may already be too late to keep it in control. We are then in the second wave.

Of course, I don't know what it will look like. I can only imagine it just like you. Will the economy collapse? Probably. Will there be like 10 x more deaths than now? Possibly. Both if we don't take into account who we truly are deep inside.

Well, then, what to do IF we were certain of such a second wave to come? I have no clue about whether some scenarios are being worked out for such a case. The super-rich are probably busy working out what to do WHEN a second wave is present. Even they should think about how to get there. The following are some ideas and suggestions in case of, say, a certainty of second wave without any miracle cure:

- The obvious. We should, of course, have no shortage in all sorts of protective means: facemasks, tracking apps, etc. At society-level, preparations may be appropriate to handle the situation.

- We should collectively avoid falling from a mental cliff into despair. That has already happened once. Relevant is not only the depth of falling but also from what height. From a substantial height, it's more hurtful, with such hurt itself fueling the whirlpool.

- We should cherish life. Many people at risk may die in isolation. They deserve more and deeper attention before that happens.

- People who work in homes for the elderly may get some additional education in handling critical conditions. Also, they may get more mental support.

- In view of economic collapse, we shouldn't spend too much money and resources that would go to waste in such a case. Many hard decisions are due.

- We should think about the balance between economic shutdown / school closures and people's lives. This will be harsher during the second wave in many countries.

- In my view, we should be open as much as possible. Does consciously deceiving people seem OK in order to get some economy going again or to let people take their vacation in a relaxed state of mind. It is still deception. It hampers the search for other solutions. It is an act of manipulation with many ramifications. Also, in this case, it may backfire economically big-time.

- From the Minding Corona viewpoint, people should be educated in the power of the mind. A denial of everything related to the deeper mind should be counterbalanced without starting a fight against anything or anyone.

- We should learn more about the positive and negative impact of the media.

- An app with relevant, immersive exercises might be translated into many languages as soon as possible.

- Some steps of Compassionate A.I. might be developed to alleviate the plight of many.

Writing some of these points feels horrible. It may be helpful to many, yet time is not on our side.

Jean-Luc Mommaerts

16. Postcoronalia – COVID complications

July 4, 2020

	Today	Total
Cases worldwide	209.028	11.182.576
Deaths worldwide	5.170	528.372

Today is the 4th of July

On a rally at Mount Rushmore, with perplexity on four stony presidential faces in the background, the US president couldn't care less for the people who seem to adore him and take pride in being led to nowhere, ramping up each other, shouting, without face masks nor social distancing. Here is a combination of everything one should not do. This also has repercussions for people worldwide. It concerns everybody.

Meanwhile, a curve from today (www.worldometers.info/coronavirus):

Daily New Cases in India

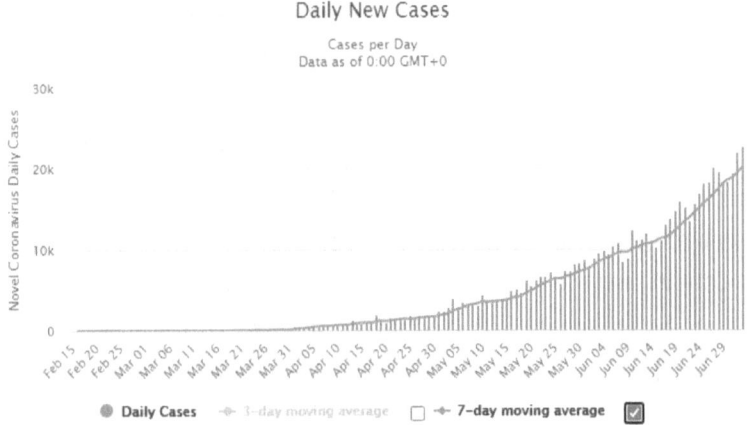

In a few weeks, India will probably – and possibly further on to a huge degree – surpass the US in its number of cases and deaths today but with little economic resilience, no access to proper healthcare for many, and no clarity about post-corona complications. The latter will be immense.

We don't know very much about postcoronalia yet.

Worldwide, more than six million coronavirus cases have officially 'recovered' to date. This number doesn't show what is meant by 'recovered.' We've barely started gaining knowledge about what happens to survivors after an episode of severe COVID. What we do know isn't encouraging. It is suspected that in the US alone as well as in Europe hundreds of thousands of people will have long-lasting symptoms after having escaped death. These symptoms may linger for months or years or even a lifetime. There will be a substantial cost at the personal level, on the healthcare system, and the economy through presenteeism (being at work but not performing at full capacity), absenteeism, and work incapacity.

Statistics focus on cases of infection and death toll. Meanwhile, little attention goes to the aftermath concerning the health of survivors. I guess this is because the news, as a mechanism, acts unidirectionally.

Diversification within a single domain dilutes the message and diminishes bait. Sorry, I'm grumpy.

Long-term symptoms and complications will be increasingly present in the news shortly. We already know that they affect many different body parts: the heart, the lungs, the liver, the brain, the endocrine-metabolic system, articulations. Dozens of articles about all of these are appearing in PubMed, the high-standard database of medical, scientific literature.

Concerning the heart and bloodstream, for instance, known complications include myocardial injury, myocarditis, acute myocardial infarction, heart failure, dysrhythmias, and venous thromboembolic events. [Long et al., 2020] Known neurological complications include headache, dizziness, myalgia, and anosmia, as well as cases of acute cerebrovascular events, encephalitis, Guillain-Barré syndrome, acute necrotizing hemorrhagic encephalopathy, and hemophagocytic lymphohistiocytosis. [Bridwell et al., 2020, Carod-Artal, 2020] Never mind the medicalese. This shows a beginning knowledge and much more to follow in the next months and years. There may also be many mild symptoms that linger without being recognized as related.

As the virus evolves in unforeseen ways, the second wave may bring more aftermath. I guess that in due time, complications will be seen everywhere in the body. Does this mean the virus reaches every part of the body? Maybe. The immune/inflammatory system does so in its overreaction, perhaps even where no viruses are present. Also, blood clotting plays a significant role, also affecting many organs.

Complications concerning the mind

After COVID-19, patients tend to have lingering symptoms of fatigue, as also happens after other viral infections. COVID-19 seems to provoke this to a higher degree and over a more extended period. Also prominent is a recurring presence of altered mental states, for example, a delusion of dying or being dead, as described from personal experience by Paul Garner, professor of infectious diseases at the Liverpool School of Tropical Medicine [BMJ, May 2020] This is especially prevalent when patients have had psychotic delirium during the acute phase. Apparently, many of these shy away from talking about it lest they be regarded as crazy, which also makes it a lonely condition.

There will probably be many cases of chronic fatigue starting right after or a while after COVID-19. The old question will turn up whether it is psychological or physical. Well, in a paradigm of body-mind unity, there is no difference. One may as well drop the battle between the two camps. The more interesting question is how to manage it. If psychological means can help in the prevention or treatment, then any misguided fighting over the distinction mainly detracts personally and at a society-level.

We can expect many survivors with PTSD (post-traumatic stress). The loneliness of many at the brink of death is unprecedented. This is even unlike wartime in which most of the dying happens at least in a sphere of togetherness. Personally, my choice regarding dying in one of both situations would be made quickly. Nevertheless, we may learn from after-war PTSD that this may appear after some time, even years after the facts. We may also learn from war-related PTSD that its management is far from evident.

Seeing PTSD as a distinct entity, there will also be more depression, phobias, OCD, etc. in survivors and relatives.

After years

It is to be expected that new physical complications will appear after many years. Time will tell, but chances are more substantial for this viral disease because of the severity of immune deregulation. This will – probably – heighten the proneness to autoimmune disorders, such as multiple sclerosis and rheumatoid arthritis. Note that the mind also plays a role in the occurrence of these.

So much more important is taking care of the mind

Properly taking the mind into account may diminish the death toll and, at the same time, the negative health consequences. Eventually, one may rightfully ask which is more important. What strikes me is that some survivors say one might as well be dead. Such utterances are not to be discarded.

According to the premise of this book, the mind is involved already from an early stage. Thus, the relief of possible complications can also start early on. One doesn't need to wait for a severe stage of illness.

What we don't know

We don't know whether a patient can be reinfected after 6 – 12 months and whether the symptoms in such cases will be less pronounced or even more. Remember that after being vaccinated for SARS-CoV, laboratory mice showed a pulmonary inflammatory overreaction when brought into contact with the living virus. [Tseng et al., 2012]

Also, people who are reinfected may have scarred lungs, heart, etc. which can make them more vulnerable. It's like being hit by the same hammer twice. Of course, these are possibilities, not certainties.

Virome

The set of commensal viruses is called the human virome, and is probably rich and diverse, although not yet very well studied because of difficulties in detecting viruses in the background of the abundant human genome, generally requiring additional manipulations. [Moore et al., 2017] Such viruses can be our guests for a long time and be prevalent, mostly causing no harm. Sometimes, they cause cancer after many years or in specific circumstances, such as immunosuppression.

The new coronavirus can become part of the virome. In that case, unfortunately, for it to become a non-dangerous element, many people will die, even years from now if no super-vaccine is developed.

The virome also shows that, in principle, viruses can be present in low numbers, escape testing (arguably), and co-start a whirlpool in specific circumstances such as seasonal and stress. This would mean that during the summer, many people can become 'test-negative carriers' with viruses present just like any other commensal. This may be happening during the summer of 2020 in Europe on a massive scale.

There is no certainty in this, but I'm completely baffled by the risk being taken.

References

[BMJ, May 2020] blogs.bmj.com/bmj/2020/05/05/paul-garner-people-who-have-a-more-protracted-illness-need-help-to-understand-and-cope-with-the-constantly-shifting-bizarre-symptoms/

[Bridwell et al., 2020] Bridwell R, Long B, Gottlieb M. Neurologic complications of COVID-19. *Am J Emerg Med*. 2020;38(7):1549.e3-1549.e7. doi:10.1016/j.ajem.2020.05.024

[Carod-Artal, 2020] Carod-Artal FJ. Neurological complications of coronavirus and COVID-19. Complicaciones neurológicas por coronavirus y COVID-19. *Rev Neurol*. 2020;70(9):311-322. doi:10.33588/rn.7009.2020179

[Long et al., 2020] Long B, Brady WJ, Koyfman A, Gottlieb M. Cardiovascular complications in COVID-19. *Am J Emerg Med*. 2020;38(7):1504-1507. doi:10.1016/j.ajem.2020.04.048

[Moore et al., 2017] Moore PS, Chang Y. Common Commensal Cancer Viruses. *PLoS Pathog*. 2017;13(1):e1006078. Published 2017 Jan 19. doi:10.1371/journal.ppat.1006078.

[Tseng et al., 2012] Tseng CT, Sbrana E, Iwata-Yoshikawa N, et al. Immunization with SARS coronavirus vaccines leads to pulmonary immunopathology on challenge with the SARS virus [published correction appears in PLoS One. 2012;7(8). doi:10.1371/annotation/2965cfae-b77d-4014-8b7b-236e01a35492]. *PLoS One*. 2012;7(4):e35421. doi:10.1371/journal.pone.0035421

17. Leadership in Corona Times

July 22, 2020

	Daily	Total
Cases worldwide	**239.113**	**15.084.963**
Deaths worldwide	**5.678**	**618.493**

Becoming Open

This chapter is targeted right within the second COVID-wave. It's a letter to the near future. With leadership, I don't mean bossy figures who tell others what to do. You might take a look at my book *Open Leadership*. This leadership is Compassionate. It takes into account the human being as a total person, far from mere-ego. We need this more than ever in times of COVID. Namely, in being genuinely, deeply oneself, one finds the Inner Strength that gives one a more direct influence also upon health-related issues that otherwise remain out of reach. This includes stress, distress, and its impact on the body in many ways, including immunologically. In short, leadership is good for health; bossiness is bad for health.

So, good leadership – which, to me, is always Open – is crucial these days. The message that goes from this to the entire population has a subconceptual influence (deep-to-deep) that is an essential tool to curb the COVID-whirlpool. Open Leadership alleviates the COVID-whirlpool just by being Open. So, the first piece of advice to leadership is to be or become Open. How? This chapter contains some suggestions.

Motivation, the Open way

Telling someone what to do is not motivation. It's like pushing a ball underwater, but this ball grows bigger and bigger. It takes an increasing amount of energy to keep the ball immersed. With less push, it comes nearer to the surface. This may heighten the pusher's conviction that more energy is needed. When the energy suddenly gets depleted, the ball breaks through the surface with a full splash. Everything is wet. That's because there was never any motivation in the first place.

All motivation is deep motivation. You need to find out what a person would do without you telling him so. You need to lead a person to what already motivates him from inside out. Easier said than done. People are not always in contact with their genuine self. For instance, one may work for a few decades, then find out that this has never been what one really wanted to do. Inner dissociation: people are living on a surface level that doesn't accord with deep-inside. As an unfortunate side effect, one may get into a groove of addictive behavior. The addiction sucks out genuine motivational energy. Many people are 'addicted' to many things – one more superficial than the other – and prone to burnout. This makes them especially vulnerable to a stress-virus that seeks this out as its niche. Something like COVID was bound to happen, and it is bound to happen again if humanity keeps following the same track.

Every communication should be oriented to being motivational. People need it not only to do what's needed but also to replenish – while doing so! – their batteries. This is a task of Open Leadership. It's what leadership should be remunerated for. Without good leadership, there is no good communication and eventually a choice only between manipulation and coercion, such as trying to 'make' people follow the social distancing rules, or sending in the COVID police and starting repression.

Face masks

We will need to wear face masks for quite some time. If we are not genuinely motivated, after a while, we will experience 'motivation fatigue.' Our incentive will dwindle. We'll even get demotivated. If demotivated, people always find reasons for not doing the right thing. This is not just a conscious process. People may really, yet incorrectly, think they are not wearing it 'for a just cause' (freedom, religion…). Look at the motivation literature: people find to a huge degree reasons that are not their true reasons. In specific experiments, subjects are led to believe that they have made a different choice than they just happened to make (one picture over another). Even more, without hesitation nor conscious awareness, the subjects concoct reasons why they think they just made the choice which they actually didn't. Likewise, people may not wear face masks for reasons that are not their genuine reasons. The main reason may be a natural dislike of blocking one's airflow, as simple as that. This complicates the matter towards letting people motivate themselves from inside. It's by far not enough to ask them about their motivations. One needs to go deeper. This can only be done through deep-to-deep communication.

Moreover, if one pushes the wrong motivational buttons, the reflex of the to-be-motivated-person is that "this reason why I should conform to the rules doesn't conform with me." The natural result is demotivation.

It is scientifically evident – not only a possibility – that other people die because of one's not wearing a mask. Look at COVID-parties. Are these youngsters not aware of that? Of course, they are. But young people need to get out their energy, dance, and do all they spontaneously do. So, are young people murderers? Of course not. They do what youngsters do if not motivated towards other behavior. Their present behavior is, of course, not correct, but the source of their behavior is correct indeed. So, if you want to quell that source, or if you don't make the right distinction between source and outcome, you are fighting against humanity and against nature itself. That is not efficient at all. So, don't look at them as murderers or as 'guilty' of anything. Instead, look at the situation as one of joint responsibility to make the best of it.

In any case, if there wouldn't have been younger generations over many generations, there would not be people. Looking at youngsters is looking at humankind. That is who we are as a species. If an older person blames a younger one for being young, he is blaming himself. Not efficient. As a leader, you should avoid stepping into these footsteps.

Instead, younger generations are to be motivated as younger generations. They can be Compassionate too, from inside out. They need motivation for that. They need to see why, as Compassion always does. Otherwise, it's mechanical. In a society in which no wisdom is respected, mostly information and data – and money, of course – older generations are readily disrespected and put aside. Why would one wear a face mask to protect them? One communication may be that this is what a Compassionate society eventually stands for. This is what makes us good people. This is what makes humankind a good species.

The fed-up-feeling

Already in May, some people had just enough of it. They didn't want to care anymore. What remained was a wanting to get out or get in: inside their mental bubble where COVID only reaches one as a distant dream from which one will awake one day. This amounts to a sheer feeling of being fed up with an unwelcome reality. It's not denial. It's not carelessness. It's a numbness, a feeling of wanting to go to a mental and moral desert where one can wait for the problems to go away miraculously, or for others to make the problems go away. It's all just too much. It's above carelessness. The caring, in a deep sense, has evaporated.

Now, in July, after a few weeks of thinking it will go better until it passes, the idea comes to an increasing number of people that it will not be over soon. Worse: perhaps the worse has yet to come. As indeed, it will. So, here's the fed-up-feeling, and that too will get stronger. A side effect is that those who try to warn for some pretty bad months readily feel hostility from those who are fed up and actively block out anything that threatens their mental bubble.

Open communication from leadership, not even necessarily deep-to-deep, but just open, may be crucial. This way, in communication, a leader may also share his feelings. If he's not open, he will not be sharing, and that shows one way or another. Thereby, the leader fails in his main leader's function: to be there as a human being and, at the same time, in his symbolic function, representing 'something higher.' That something higher is many things, above all else the real symbol, which is hard to comprehend. It also includes the representation of the group as a team. Members of the team look at the leader to mold their expectations, sometimes even their feelings. Without team-feeling, people may be like projectiles being thrown through the air until being fed up. A leader brings people together, not just in words but truly, and enables them to trust each other and the group as a whole. Working together, the future will be a success. This is necessary within open communication.

Without this open communication, trust will vanish. Guiding people like puppets on a string is short-lived. The puppets lose momentum until there is none left. Contrary to this, open communication shows trustworthiness. One may show one's doubt; no problem in that. A boss thrives on certainty, not a leader. A leader shows how he tries to make the best of it for all people concerned. That includes doubt. In this, as in many things, bossiness grows out of a relative lack of leadership. There is no blame for things past, but a responsibility towards the future.

If possible, an 'enemy' should be avoided. In the case of the virus, the enemy is readily chosen. Such enemy-picking is the easiest way out of genuine leadership. It also communicates aggression and is this way, before you know it, one more element in the COVID-whirlpool. Uniting people because of the unison itself is much more positive. Therefore, it is much better to avoid all talk about 'fighting the virus, defeating the virus, killing the virus.' The virus is, strictly seen, not even alive. Moreover, if fighting happens in an individual case of disease, what is being fought against is the patient himself. Who can think that this doesn't play a role at the subconceptual pattern level? It may do so to a life-threatening degree.

Stress can profoundly change people.

People react differently when under severe stress. Everybody may have had such experiences at oneself or others. A Compassionate way is to accept this and make the best of it. In times of corona, this may play a huge role, which is obvious to anyone who lives it. People may react more short-tempered. There is more misunderstanding, more aggression, more egotism, narrowness, survival instinct. It's harder to be Compassionate. This can deteriorate in a vicious circle. A political manipulator may abuse this for personal gains or even simply out of post-traumatic revenge. A leader is needed to prevent this.

Leadership, stress, and burnout are deeply related to each other. Open Leadership alleviates stress within a population. This may not be readily visible in individual cases. Yet, it can have an abundance of influence upon many personal lives. These people are not necessarily grateful because they don't necessarily see where it comes from. On the other hand, contented people make a society that is as friendly to the leader as the leader is to the people. The ancient Chinese had a strong opinion about this. For them, the well-being of the empire and all citizens was dependent on the way of the leader, perhaps most of all in an invisible, non-dualistic (= subconceptual) sense. This points to non-conscious processing, and Openness in Leadership. At least, the intuition was very much alive. This is relevant in times of corona. We all need such leadership now, independently of whether the political system is a democracy or a one-party system.

Aurelis app + Lisa

A bold statement: when everybody uses this app, the whirlpool does not 'take hold' in many individuals, nor in large groups. To divulge it as widely as possible, the app is made available for free. In my view, it should be given attention to by all. There are many lives to be saved. The background for this app is one of body-mind-unity and trust in one's inner strength from inside out. Culturally, these are not evident. Many people, including physicians, live and work in another mind frame and thus may experience difficulty in accepting the app's efficiency. That is very much a pity. The result in human suffering is tremendous on many levels, in many domains. Looked upon from a future perspective, it's mindboggling.

With Lisa (A.I.-driven coach-bot), the whirlpool may even turn the other way. People can be approached individually and as efficiently as possible. Mental exercises can be molded on a personal basis. Moreover, with real-world evidence research, Lisa can be continually enhanced, as well as scientifically investigated. This is a future I wish to be in.

18. Corona: Super-Stress, Super-Spreading?

July 26, 2020

	Daily	Total
Cases worldwide	257.789	16.189.203
Deaths worldwide	5.689	647.574

On top of an influence on COVID-progression, does stress also influence the rate of infection by infected persons? In that case, can the AURELIS-app diminish this rate?

Super-spreading

Some viral-infected people spread the virus more than others. This has been found in many infectious diseases, including in salmonellosis, tuberculosis, SARS-1 (2003) and MERS (2015). An 80-20 rule may be applicable. More or less, 20% of the infected people provoke 80% of new infections. According to some studies, even much less provokes much more. The definition of super-spreader is vague The term is used to denote people who are at the high end of the curve of infectivity. An extreme case is a person in South Korea, known only as patient 31, who transmitted the virus to over 1,100 people at an early stage of the outbreak. [https://graphics.reuters.com/CHINA-HEALTH-SOUTHKOREA-CLUSTERS/0100B5G33SB/index.html]

This is crucial. If we know what makes a person into a super-spreader, we can see how to diminish their infectivity, and, for that sake, the infectivity of anyone. This way, we can probably solve a substantial part of the problem in the best way: by preventing it.

Relevant factors in super-spreading are described as related to viral characteristics, personal behavior, and environment. Behavior (nonchalance) and environment (sports venues, churches, business, even hospitals) are rather evident. As an example, in the news these days, US federal agents in Portland, Oregon use teargas on shouting protesters (mainly protesting against the agents), drive them together, confine them in vans, stress them in many other ways. Absurd.

Where's the stress?

Meanwhile, after reading all previous chapters of this book, what we are missing in the research is psychosocial stress. I did an extensive search in PubMed today and found nothing corona-related in humans.

As to bats, I found on the Internet a communication by Prof. Vikram Misra, a veterinary microbiologist from the University of Saskatchewan [https://news.usask.ca/media-release-pages/2018/stressed-bats-can-increase-spread-of-deadly-viruses-.php] :

> "Bats have a really benign relationship with their viruses until you stress them through secondary infections or other stressors… That's when they start producing and shedding more viruses." What' other stressors' may be, is not clear in this communication. Elsewhere on the same page, we find: "Bats are responding to stress from such things as habitat destruction, lack of nutrition and infections by increasing the production and shedding of viruses that cause serious and often fatal diseases in humans and other animals."

Hmm. Not much. On another page, we find from the same:

> "When a bat experiences stress to their immune system, it disrupts this immune system-virus balance and allows the virus to multiply." And interestingly: "We see that

the MERS coronavirus can very quickly adapt itself to a particular niche... Coronaviruses rapidly adapt to the species they infect." That's including us.

In conclusion, science doesn't help in this respect. Disappointing, I dare say. We know nothing. That, of course, doesn't show there is nothing to know. It only shows that anything is possible. The possible range for the importance of psychological factors in infectivity is from nothing to huge. Our tool in order to find some guidance is common sense.

Common sense

If the immune system has trouble subduing an invader (bacterium, virus), logically, the pathogenic load will increase. In COVID-19, no exception, a higher viral load means more infectivity. From this and the whole present book until now, we can deduce that, most probably, stress plays a substantial role in infectivity. With present-day technology, this is difficult to prove in the human case. In animals such as mice, sorry for the mice, such experiments can be done. I would love – sorry for the mice, again! – to see them done.

Coronaviruses seem to adapt well to their host. In a way, this is not different to other viruses such as Influenza. In the latter case, in the pandemic years from 1918 onwards, the Influenza-virus adapted by way of not killing too many people. Not stupid, because: no host, no replication of the virus itself. So, over very many of its short-lived generations, the virus became less virulent. Even so, people are still dying from continually mutated viral strains. But as a stress-virus, SARS-CoV-2 is different in that it lets itself be replicated and shedded during days of little immune reaction (weak phase). When this flops to over-reaction (hard phase), the virus already doesn't need us anymore. Super-spreaders have super-spread it around.

Well, that's the picture. I'm sure that future insights will show this not to be of the utmost accuracy. We will learn to refine this and take some errors out. Even so, the mainline is probably correct. As a consequence, we should take this at heart to an immense degree.

The Aurelis app?

[see: "Free App to Relieve COVID"]

In that case, and turning to the Aurelis app, which is available meanwhile in the app stores, I absolutely recommend to use it from the first symptoms or COVID-positivity onwards. In that case, the reason why is twofold:

- helping yourself to stay or get out of the COVID-whirlpool as well as possible, relieving sickness, complications, and a chance to die
- helping others through making oneself less infectious

Regarding the latter, I think of an immune system that may be turned on more readily, shortening the period in which the virus can run around the body ad libitum and heighten its viral load, and shedding. I also think of less coughing and sneezing and running around in distress. Dear reader, I don't know about you, but personally, I can orient my attention to my lower airways at any time and start feeling some irritation, up to coughing – not simulating to cough – out of nowhere. I guess this is a self-influence that anybody can exert, if not always equally consciously initiated.

If the rate of infectivity drops, fewer people die. If more infected people recuperate, fewer people die. It is as simple as that.

19. The Virus is Not the Enemy

July 29, 2020

	Today	Total
Cases worldwide	247.581	16.883.793
Deaths worldwide	5.567	662.481

This goes further upon Chapter 7, written three months and half a million official COVID deaths ago.

The virus side

The virus is just a piece of RNA that wears a coating when outside of the living cells that it uses as hosts for viral replication. Is a piece of RNA an enemy? It doesn't choose to hurt anyone, of course. It doesn't have the ability to choose.

Or one can look at the virus as the conglomerate of all COVID-viruses together. After all, a human body is also a conglomerate of many tiny elements, our body cells. In that sense, there is more complexity. Whereas a simple piece of RNA is more a mechanism than a living being, the whole may be seen more readily as living. It's even more living than each of us, human beings, since it's almost immortal. Long after all the presently living humans are dead, the virus will still be alive in our offspring. Moreover, this one whole viral being is intelligent in some sense. It adapted rashly to a new host, us, and is still adjusting. We don't know at what rate, but the thought is scary. Now, this whole being doesn't see us as a friend, only as a mechanism for creating its progeny. Also, it doesn't see us as very intelligent. It finds its ways quite easily, as the numbers show. There is indeed something of an enemy in all this. Its intelligence is 'brute force learning;' in other words: pure trial and error. That's smart enough to keep thriving in competition with human intelligence.

The metaphor side

Calling the virus 'the enemy' has, in most cases, other connotations. Fighting the virus, defeating the enemy, killing the virus, getting it on its knees. It seems just a way of talking, but there is frequently more than meets the ear in a way of talking. Enemy-talk conjures up images of aggression, anxiety, and them-the-enemy. At present, huge populations are inoculated with this fodder for the COVID-whirlpool. In that sense, it's a substantial part of the problem. I would recommend finding another metaphor. Scaring people with war-talk into following the rules shows a lack of leadership. It's bad for health.

A science exists about the use of metaphors in human speech as part of critical discourse analysis. (*) In this, language is seen as part of the way that people seek to promote particular views of the world and naturalize them. It can reveal political, ideological, or cultural investment. It shows underlying assumptions. It can be powerful in deep communication. Language not only describes the world but co-models the concepts with which people build a world of perceptions and interpretations that then forms the subjective world we live in.

In a worst-case, the war metaphor can be abused by a manipulator. In wartime, people tend to rally behind a savior who promises to protect them or at least be their unitor against the enemy. The 'leader' becomes the symbol for the group in a negative and possibly catastrophic sense. This doesn't need to be consciously concocted by the manipulator. It's enough for him to follow the underlying cultural stream that leads him there. For this, there needs to be this underlying stream. I'm afraid it is streaming hard nowadays. The reason for this is simple: much cultural-technological change without proper guidance or leadership. Thus comes lousy leadership, a harder flowing stream, and a whirlpool now and then.

Culture includes medicine. The present-day war against the virus is happening in the context of medicine of war: diseases are the enemy, medications the weapons, and doctors the heroes in combat. Unfortunately, present-day medicine is beset with psycho-somatics, in which fighting the disease equals fighting the patient. These are harsh words that I substantiate thoroughly in *Your Mind as Cure*. People should urgently learn to appreciate the mind and its power to get sick as well as to heal in many ways. How we fell into this rut of self-depreciation is a long story of money, status, and power (bad leadership). Anyway, at present, this same rut is followed concerning the virus. It's not new. It's a strongly flowing stream. I encounter quite a few people who feel this, yet let themselves flow along for egotistic sake. That's too bad. In my view, the future mainly depends on them — even their own future, and surely that of their children.

In viral enemy metaphor, I see an idea of conceptual (misguided) righteousness in a mortal battle against … what exactly? Delving deeper, are we getting here at something telling about the core of a much wider human problem, being distress related in the broadest sense?

What are we precisely fighting against?

The all too human side

At present, in Belgium and especially in Antwerp, where I am writing this text, we see a strong upsurge of cases. As a consequence, we are witnessing a second lockdown. To make things softer, we call it a soft lockdown. Great. In several ways, it's harsher than ever before, probably in an attempt to save the economy. At the start of this book, I wrote about getting angry when this would happen. I am angry now, and will probably be even more. On paper, that is. Rest assured, I keep my friendliness. What strikes me, though, is a different atmosphere, a different look in people's eyes. There is an enemy in the air, a possible enemy in any encounter. This is according to the metaphor. Anyone can be infected and contagious. Anyone can carry the enemy. Thus, looking at anyone, you might be looking at the enemy. People themselves become each other's enemy. I would say eventually, but I see it happening now.

In enemy setting and quite dystopically presented, the virus attacks people, of whom some get severely ill, probably the 'weak and vulnerable.' Many people deem themselves not to be weak. They resist the idea of themselves as being weak, so they defy the enemy by not taking care. The weak ones are, well, the other ones. In the US – and to some degree in other parts of the world – this also becomes a partisan issue. "Don't be weak!" is like a seldom outspoken, underlying slogan. Weak (or a bit stupid) is the other side of the aisle. Even more, if you are at the correct side of the aisle and you do succumb to the disease, then something is probably wrong with you. You are, deep down, one of the weak. You don't belong to those worthy of thriving. Then the virus becomes part of nature doing its job in a Malthusian way of the worst kind.

In this dystopic narrative, people are supposed to be careless warriors, oblivious of their own health, and that of anyone else, as a way to filter out the weak. Defiance itself (no mask, no social distancing) becomes an act of bravery. The virus, being invisible, helps in this regard. Hospitalized patients are also invisible, not "part of us," because "we are the strong ones." The enemy is not only the virus anymore, but also the weak ones at the other side, and even within the own ranks. At the same time and from the other side, the enemy is not only the virus anymore, but also the incomprehensibly careless ones.

This dystopia is not my kind of world. How to resist it: by being rational while valuing human depth. I think this is not just my way. It is the only way. Thus, it is a fundamental choice. Fighting against the enemy is not part of this choice, even while being regarded as 'either enemy or foe.' The latter is divisive. Within the war metaphor itself, if the virus could laugh, it would be shaking its belly.

I know this is thin ice. I might fall through it. On the other side, many people might fall through the ice, not necessarily virus-related. Meanwhile, it's worthwhile to learn how to skate.

The immune side

COVID is a psycho-somatic condition. This means that looking at it from a psychological (mainly subconceptual) viewpoint is as worthy and effective as looking at it from a physical perspective. The best way lies in a combination of both. The mind is as powerful as the virus.

Because of this, the war metaphor may do much damage. Note the returning idea within this book: At first, the virus attacks on the basis of a weakened immune system. This is weakened through much chronic stress of many origins, with on top the acute/subacute stress from what is happening to the world, one's immediate environment, and oneself. The viral enemy takes advantage of this. From the start on, it takes advantage of the COVID-whirlpool for a multiplication of effectiveness. The whirlpool, one can say, is part of the niche to which the virus has adapted very well. This is the consequence of a long-term evolution and a short-term coincidence.

Then the immune system flops into a hard stance. The heavy guns are taken out of the warehouse. The shooting is done with little discrimination. Much of one's own tissue gets destroyed. The patient may suffer more from this war-like overreaction than from the direct enemy maneuvers. Now, to what degree can a war metaphor influence such immune reactions? The future will tell. Probably to a diverse degree, relatively seen and in most people. In an absolute sense, it may push many beyond the brink of survival. This way, it becomes crucial.

Meanwhile, the fighting metaphor makes us prone to forget ourselves as part of causality. In a few years, using A.I. and real-world evidence science, we will be able to look much better into such issues. For the moment, there is a huge domain of the unknown and many indications of psychological influences upon the immune system that would astonish many outsiders. Moreover, when the virus comes to vaccinated people, we may hope the interaction doesn't lead to deadly eosinophilic pneumonia. Focusing too much on the virus-as-enemy, we might forget that this is a real possibility.

The side of human suffering

This historic period brings mental suffering to many people in much broader ways than what is directly virus- and immune-related. Especially those who were already suffering before are having a hard time. I see them as the sensitive ones who, without proper support, are at risk of becoming the vulnerable ones. Also, I see an immense lack of proper support. Worldwide, many of the vulnerable are to be found within the ranks of the defiant ones in an attempt to find solace and protection by showing off, until the armor breaks.

This is part of the COVID-whirlpool, in which all kinds of stress come together with the virus. Scaring people into social distancing is improper, let alone a curfew, as imposed in Antwerp today for the first time since WWII. Meanwhile, sales-shopping goes on for the sake of the economy. Here lies a breakdown of rationality and leadership.

The war metaphor brings additional anxiety and aggression. The enemy is to be feared and fought against. The weak will fare badly. The cause of much suffering lies in auto-aggression or – as I like to call it – inner dissociation. This way, heightening an atmosphere of aggression and war makes people prone to dissociate even further and get caught in a bubble of mere-ego. [See *The Journey Towards Compassionate A.I.*] The virus-as-enemy metaphor is a huge disservice to many and, eventually, to society as a whole.

The postcoronalia side

This is about the complications after being severely ill. The patient has been defeated by the enemy, almost mortally wounded. I hope that many people in postcoronalia are led to using their inner strength at this stage. Inner strength is not a fluffy concept. It is what can be achieved with the use of autosuggestion and subconceptual processing/communication. There is much science about this, so much that not taking it into account should, nowadays, be seen as the non-scientific way to proceed. The clock has remained the same, but the hand has progressed.

Given the massive immune disturbances that we see happening in COVID, there will be a lot of postcoronalia. What we can expect is, among other things:

- Depression: prevalent in patients during and after periods of systemic inflammation. There is probably a two-way influence between depression and inflammation. Both are substantially mediated by the central nervous system.

- Autoimmune disorders (multiple sclerosis, rheumatic arthritis...): also being related to other viral infections, sometimes after many years. New flare-ups are, without any remaining doubt, related to preceding episodes of heightened stress. The psyche is definitely involved.

To diminish the chances of these and other chronic illnesses after COVID, these patients should be supported accordingly from at least the moment they enter the hospital with COVID symptoms. I would also recommend it to those who put themselves or have been put in quarantine. Massive immune reactions may be prevented or relieved, thus also postcoronalia. When complications arrive, of course, all possible support should be given conceptually and subconceptually. Completely discarding one or both is bad medicine.

Fighting for

We are fighting for a better world. The virus is not the enemy but just a part of the environment in which the struggle goes on. It's not a struggle against, but for, as in an excellent judo competition.

Let's fight for a world in which humans can work together as much as possible to counter this mishap that has befallen us. Let's search for a medication that stops the replication of the virus. Let's not forget our fundamental human values. Let's learn about ourselves as much as possible through this ordeal, to make it worthwhile after all. Let's have an eye for every person dying from COVID, and indeed also from complications on the medical or economic level. For instance, in the developing world, many children are at risk of dying from a lack of food and clean water as a result of necessary lockdowns. Let's care for them too, even if the rich man's money has dwindled. Let's learn together how to prevent the next pandemic. Let's try to find a vaccine that shields us like a sun blocker shields us from negative sunrays.

Note that none of this is a fighting metaphor. A shield metaphor may be better if not being brought to war again. There is no weakness in shielding. One may shield oneself from the sun. We don't fight the sun. We may shield this planet from incoming big meteors. We may shield the next generations from paying the price for our silly conduct. We may shield ourselves from the virus.

We don't have to fight against the virus. It would be much better not to.

(*) A good book about this is *How to Do Critical Discourse Analysis: A Multimodal Introduction* by David Machin and Andrea Mayr.

20. Autumn of COVID: Disaster² Already?

July 29, 2020

	Today	Total
Cases worldwide	290.459	17.177.560
Deaths worldwide	7.036	669.572

(Re-)emergence

COVID (re-)emerges in all kinds of countries where strict measures have not been maintained. This includes countries where the virus has never well receded (such as the US), countries where it has not peaked before (such as parts of Australia), and countries that saw a huge decrease after disaster (such as Spain and Belgium). Everywhere, the virus is waiting for a chance, while not waiting for humans to be ready. The COVID-virus doesn't reward previous efforts.

We don't see Influenza flaring up now. Influenza is seasonal. Does this mean that COVID is not seasonal? The most pertinent question concerning the near future in Europe and the US: Will COVID flare up in the autumn on top of what we see now? The answer, as far as I can see, is: of course. While autumn is not yet the big Influenza/Corona period of the year – which is wintertime – COVID shows to be more infective and lethal than Influenza. That doesn't mean it's less seasonal.

Seasonality + Lethality => Disaster²?

We will be taken by surprise, apparently, again. This time, we should know better. I see many people and companies, organizations, and politicians act as if we know 'the enemy' by now, and are better prepared than earlier this year for what's coming.

But in a way, we are not. As mentioned, the fact that the virus can surge in the summer doesn't mean it will hit less in autumn. I see this deduction being made, but it's logically just plain wrong. It probably means that the virus will hit *even harder* in the autumn and beyond.

Of course, we are better prepared for something like what happened from March 2020 onwards. The problem is: what is coming is different in two respects: People are even less mentally ready (being tired, sad, horrified, bored, burned out, demotivated), and the virus may hit harder because, among other things, lockdown is economically seen even less evident. On top of these, the COVID-whirlpool [see: "Covid Whirlpool"] will take us towards new territory without us knowing what is happening. This new territory within the whirlpool is made up by ourselves, as well as by the virus. It will be surprising once more mainly because of its subconceptual nature. Thus:

- We think we can take this challenge as a linear process, building up defenses.
- The reality will be exponential again.

Humanity has seldom experienced a lack of arrogance. The accompanying disillusion will become another part of the whirlpool. Now, we think we are intelligent enough to 'control the beast just by putting more conceptual defense on top of defense.' If needed, we build the wall higher. That may be OK in many circumstances, but not if something comes flying over the wall. A simple wall – as a construction of bricks – doesn't suffice. We need to use our subconceptual wings. See previous chapters/blog texts. Without them, we get into disaster².

Do I seem to be promoting my idea that the subconceptual level is crucial in the COVID happening? As much as I would like to be wrong in prediction, from the health-related side, there is little chance. My opinion is based on many elements and robust synthesis. Virologists are medical specialists in half of the matter. I am a specialist in the other half. No bird flies on one wing.

Seasonality means that we should do whatever we can to get the numbers much lower over the summer in order to be able to keep them down through the autumn. During the summer, we could get them to near zero. That would be a position from which we can do the necessary to keep them so, relatively, for a while. Contrary to this, if we glide towards autumn with already higher numbers, the whirlpool turbo will make us lose control before we can say w.h.i.r.l.p.o.o.l.

Good, bad, ugly

I have a Ph.D. in mind-body medical science, not in economics. My view from the latter side is limited. I try to put together in a scheme what strikes me as relevant. That is, from a helicopter view, not much.

The good	The bad
Remdesivir	No vaccine yet
Immunoglobulins	Medications relieve only slightly.
Dexamethasone	
Anticoagulants and other support	Snotty children – and adults
Face masks are available.	Post-traumatic + new stress
They also protect against other viruses.	We may need better face masks.
Contact tracing	Problems with contact tracing
Social distancing, hand cleaning	Less money available
Many businesses are better prepared.	The economy demands human contacts.

We (should) react more quickly.   People may get complacent.

Many people are fed up.

The ugly

COVID-whirlpool +++

Again, we don't see this coming.

It may be (much) harsher.

What I don't mention in the scheme, because it's very uncertain, is the possibility of viral mutations. Also, economically, there may be more critical elements. This is going to cost another few trillion, if not the entire economy and world peace. Of course, the very rich will rebound. On top of this, it will take a lot of professional lives and livelihoods. For instance, fitness centers, bars, and restaurants will most probably not remain open for more than a few weeks this year. Mass gatherings will not be possible, let alone advisable, in the autumn nor winter time. Other sectors will surely be hit hard too. Economists may know what this means to the treasury, banks, and people's money. More pending foreclosures are still due to the consequences of the first wave. This adds to the whirlpool.

Taking yourself seriously

As a human being, you have a lot inside that has not been explored, let alone put to proper usage. We could use this well in the present situation. However, a basic cultural stream prevents most people from doing so. This makes them dependent. What they are dependent on (people, organizations, cultural ideas even) profits from this situation. This doesn't mean that it's necessarily done with conscious insight. It's a mechanism, used in many places, together forming a stream with strong current and in which individual people flow along. This stream's sturdy current makes some people misinterpret a flowing along with it as strength, a standing strong against it as weakness. Moreover, there is sometimes aggression involved, such as from some who flow in this stream towards those who don't. This makes some people see an enemy where is none, and a friend where is really the foe. Guess what happens. The future will be created by a transcendence – or lack – of this. It's a time in which the free and the brave can stand up.

Yes, taking yourself seriously is a worthy cause. It doesn't necessarily bring money or status. It brings worthiness. I hope this remains valuable to many. I know it will be more valuable in the future. I have been exploring it – what I call *Inner Strength* – for quite a few years now. On one of my vagrancies, I have made an in-depth analysis of human being in this regard and described it in *The Journey Towards Compassionate A.I.*

What have I done?

Too little. The Aurelis app is now available [see: "Free App to Relieve COVID"]. A.I. enhancements are possible, including Lisa [see: "Lisa"]. Other developments, translations, visibility, connections, B2B cooperation, etc. are appropriate. The app can be made more encompassing.

I have written and am writing this book and others, available at Amazon. It all lacks good marketing, due to a continually being stuck in a catch-22 of finances and possibilities. As a feeble excuse, I can point out that a basic cultural stream as I just described doesn't allow for the usual marketing efforts to be successful in the countercurrent direction. The stream honors what flows in the course of the stream itself. Especially tricky is the fact that it's hardly visible and yet pervades everything. This is typical for broadly distributed patterns. It's why people don't always change easily, and cultures also don't change easily. On the positive side, when a change is finally realized, it's quite stable.

Legacy

If we don't collectively take action, I look with horror at a preventable disaster[2]. Without a concerted effort, it will sadly be stuff for a detailed postscript to MINDING CORONA. Then this text becomes a legacy of what could have been, dated midsummer 2020. In a few years, using A.I. means and real-world evidence, a proof of what is happening (either or not realized) in the undercurrent will be possible. There is no doubt in my mind. I would like to take part in this and intend to give it my best shot. At present, we 'only' have more than enough stringent cues, no directly COVID-related experimental science – which would not be possible right now and with the usual means. Anyone who cares to think about this with a straight mind carries responsibility.

———————

As a physician in matter, I also have just a few recommendations that I don't encounter elsewhere; for what it's worth:

- I recommend, with caution, the use of small doses of acetylsalicylic acid (Aspirin) when in quarantine. Of course, this needs to be scientifically investigated. I found one article in 'Medical Hypotheses.' That's it. Without contra-indication, the use of 50 mg daily cannot harm. I'd rather see it as a preventive measure of physical support instead of an additional medical weapon.

- When running past someone outside and without a mask, closing your mouth is recommended, diminishing the spread of viruses. Every little bit helps.

- Not talking loudly in company is better. When on a bus, for instance, it will probably make a difference.

- Follow the rules, mindlessly perhaps. OK, that said, try to motivate yourself – and others – first. Following rules on top of motivation is different. There is mind involved.

- Carry the Aurelis app on your smartphone. The sheer thought that it's there may act like a placebo. In my view, placebo is quite mindless. Besides, in due time, you might think of applying it and come to appreciate it.

21. How to Make Someone Take His Vaccination

July 31, 2020

	Today	Total
Cases worldwide	**289.414**	**17.752.916**
Deaths worldwide	**6.430**	**682.393**

A little story of long ago

At 23 years of age, I went to Brazil for a few months to do medical work in a favela (shantytown) of Salvador Da Bahia. Ow, impressionable youth! As part of my documentation, I read a book about medics in the tropics. One story in this book was meant as an admonition for caution. I never checked the truth of the story, but I remember it, just as you will. In a village – somewhere – well-meaning Western doctors performed a vaccination campaign on all children. A few weeks later, they came back to check the results. To their horror, they encountered carnage. The medicine man of the village had ordered the villagers to 'cut out the vaccines.' Need I write more?

Many people object to vaccinations in science-ridden US and Europe as well as in a small tropical village harboring a witch doctor. The morale of the little story was that the Western doctors were blatantly at fault for not listening better to the indigenous people.

Listen. Don't think you are correct before everyone thinks more or less the same correctness. That's a challenging but necessary job. Of course, you may be 100% conceptually accurate. That's not good enough. Ask the children.

The problem

Dr. A. Fauci, in a congress hearing today, is cautiously optimistic that a vaccine will come this year. Let's also be cautious. With all that I know about what I don't know – being a lot – my intuition tells me that a suitable vaccine will be there (in the US) by the beginning of 2021. From that date, over the following year, most Americans will be able to get a vaccine. Many will not want one. Same scenario in Europe. Problematic.

How to make someone take his vaccination

First of all, I would say, by making it *his* vaccination, not *your* vaccination. Remember always that you want an excellent end-result, not a good feeling of superiority amid much suffering. You are a Compassionate person.

Me too. So, I went for guidance to the WHO website and a few others. I read about the reasons why people don't want to be vaccinated or let their children be vaccinated. I also encounter the reasons why most of these reasons are bad. Succinctly, we can see as anti-vax reasons:

- **Philosophical objections**: such as to government interference into what they believe should be a personal choice
- **Religious beliefs**: note that there is still no foolproof vaccine against witchcraft, even in Belgium
- Concerns about safety: potential allergic reactions; illness after vaccination, parents citing many medical risks, including autism by some mercury-based preservative (Thimerosal), as potential consequences of being vaccinated, fear of 'hot lots' of vaccine with more adverse events and deaths, possible long-term effects

we don't even know about, multiple vaccinations at the same time increasing the risk of harmful side effects

- **Concerns about efficacy**: the flu vaccine not protecting against all strains of the flu, people still getting the disease after vaccination, a belief that diseases were disappearing or have been eliminated due to better sanitation and hygiene, not vaccines

- **Mistrust**: of the government, of pharmaceutical companies who want to sell a product regardless of harmful consequences, of poorly understood science or unknown chemicals, preferring 'natural' or homeopathic treatments instead.

As the remedy, I encountered this basic admonition for well-meaning Western doctors: "Most of the concerns that create opposition to vaccination are misconceptions. Therefore, make sure people have accurate information with which to make an informed decision." That is indeed very true. Also, it is the easy job.

After this comes the hard work of motivation.

We sincerely believe that the FDA and other scientific approval agencies do their job in perfect seriousness. We want to eradicate COVID from the planet. Since that is, of course, not possible, we want, at least, a situation of as little casualties as possible.

It is necessary to not only listen to the vaccine-reluctants, but really very well Listen to them. To understand and motivate someone, you need to mentally overlap. You need to make the other's argument into yours, of course, while keeping your wits and common sense. That is not an easy thing to do. With some exercise, one can get better at it. Just make sure you don't lose yourself in reality. It's like watching an excellent movie that can take you to a different place and time for a while.

What you can accomplish then is not a miracle, of course. But it's not nothing either, even when you don't see any immediate turnaround. One important – not so visible – effect is that, through your Listening, you enable the other person to move a bit. It's like when you want to move a big car, and you push and push and then suddenly it starts to move a bit.

It's just a tiny bit but a crucial one. If you support the other person from inside, and he keeps on pushing at himself, and others don't obstruct, it's going to work. It may even be the only way it can durably work.

Some elements

For instance, a lack of trust in science will not diminish through sheer scientific argumentation. It may even get worse, and, of course, you do not want that. So, don't do that. Of course, scientific argumentation is still important, but not so much as to the argumentation itself. It's more important in the way you bring it. You might keep this in mind: science is meaningful to you because it means something to you. The same applies to the other person.

I believe in the importance of Compassion. Someone else may believe in Jehovah. This is a case of one belief to another, not of one belief to none. In-depth, this is crucial. It brings us on equal footage. We can argue on the same level. I can search for Compassion in the other's belief and ask respect for mine. This might even help; who knows?

Those who fear that vaccinations causes autism live in a challenging world with danger on several sides. They may cognitively distance themselves from rational argumentation to relieve some of the stress. What would you do in the other's place? Would you push your dear one into autism? It's difficult. It's interesting. The best you can do is try to understand profoundly before sending the army. The same for other medical risks in which you don't believe. What the scientific community could do, meanwhile, is tackle issues such as autism from a more encompassing viewpoint, taking a non-dualistic, thus realistic, view on the human being. That would save the day, the century, and humanity from much unnecessary suffering. We don't need less science. We need more.

To mitigate some bias, I think it's better to not talk about vaccine or no-vaccine, but about the *state of being vaccinated*. That way, one compares two states. One can, rightfully, say that the state of being vaccinated – while carrying some risk – carries FAR LESS risk than the state of not being vaccinated. That brings the balance in better perspective. It brings motivation not in a for-versus-against, but in a for-versus-for. Even the concrete numbers can be put in the scales at both sides. This way, there is no fight against anti-vaxxers, but a continuous joint effort to find the best' for.' In this effort, you can show your concern as much as you like. At least, it will not make matters worse.

Note that I didn't start this text with statistics, but with a powerful story that, in a way, I can emotionally bring in relation to me, showing my emotions and asking for yours. That took your attention enough to read on to this point, didn't it?

Apart from the given reasons, may a vaccine also have a symbolic meaning to many people? There is a combination of coercion and ingestion or injection. People feel forced to take it. A vaccine is unique in this. The individual feels invaded by society. The former is personal, the latter impersonal. People associate this with the theft of freedom, especially in the West. It's more than about taking away something. It's about an invasion of integrity, a symbolic theft of individuality.

Some more COVID vaccine related questions

Big pharma will gain big money. Shares are sky-rocketing already. People see and wonder: are these companies Compassionate? Really? I hear in congress (on screen) that vaccinations will be dispersed at production cost. Hmm, year after year? I don't think so. Read the small letters. So, with an expensive vaccine from 2022 onwards, will most non-anti-vaxxers buy it? Will they not feel deceived? Will this not create a backlash?

I wonder what the plans are for children and youth who don't get sick but are infective. Will they all happily get their shots for the sake of Methuselahs like me? And if they don't, what must we do?

All in all, with cautious certainty, I guess that vaccines can solve around 40% of the COVID health problem in developed countries. That would be nice. What about the rest of the world population?

I have a nightmare

The vaccine exit will not be miraculous. We will have this virus on our back and in our lungs for a long time. Herd immunity will not be reachable. The virus will not attenuate as other viruses do after a period of rampaging. This one has found a niche in which it doesn't need to attenuate. All it needs is enough of us.

Of course, humanity will survive and learn to live with the situation. I hope, in a Compassionate way.

22. Only 'Control' + COVID-Whirlpool = DISASTER

August 1, 2020

	Today	Total
Cases worldwide	**255.811**	**18.008.699**
Deaths worldwide	**5.601**	**688.016**

[see also: "The Future of the COVID Story"]

I am a medical doctor, specialized in mind-body medicine, master in cognitive science and A.I. The reason I start with this is that my expertise is absolutely pertinent, on par with, and complementary to the expertise of virologists. So, I wrote a book, made an app. Here is theory and practice, available to all, for free, financed by me. Together, it can help tremendously. [see: "Free App to Relieve COVID"]

I contacted virologists, nationally and internationally, several times. They stay at home in their silo of expertise. That's understandable, but meanwhile, the situation is dramatic worldwide, and the really big disaster is yet to come. A year from now, that will be all too apparent. It's better to come out of the ivory tower now, of course, while not getting stuck in an unscientific swamp. For every scientific-minded person, there is a responsibility in doing so. I guess that includes you. Note that as to mind-body-unity medicine, I AM a full-fledged scientific expert, arguably one of the best documented in the world. Still, the message is a difficult one to divulge.

If you want to cooperate in any way, please contact me. You can easily find enough documentation in my writings (LinkedIn posts, AURELIS blogs, books on Amazon) and developments for an informed decision. For an introduction, written in May, you can read Minding COVID: a Different Story. This blog-text is also an appendix of my book about it.

Only 'control'

The five measures of 'control' as promoted also by the US CDC:

- wash your hands
- social distancing (+/- 6 feet, 1.5 m)
- stay at home
- wear a face mask
- avoid touching your face

Absolutely. This, together, is one wing of the bird. No bird flies on one wing. The measures are necessary, but not enough. The reason is that nobody performs them perfectly and, without a dystopic dictatorship, too many people will perform them only to a so-so degree. Just look around. There is a lot of mishap, even in summer. Winter will be much worse.

The bird needs two wings.

The second is our own human mind. I still don't see this being discussed in any relevant way in the management of COVID. That is, not in cause;, only in consequence does mind-stuff seem to be important. While, of course, it is very much part of the COVID-whirlpool as summarized in this diagram:

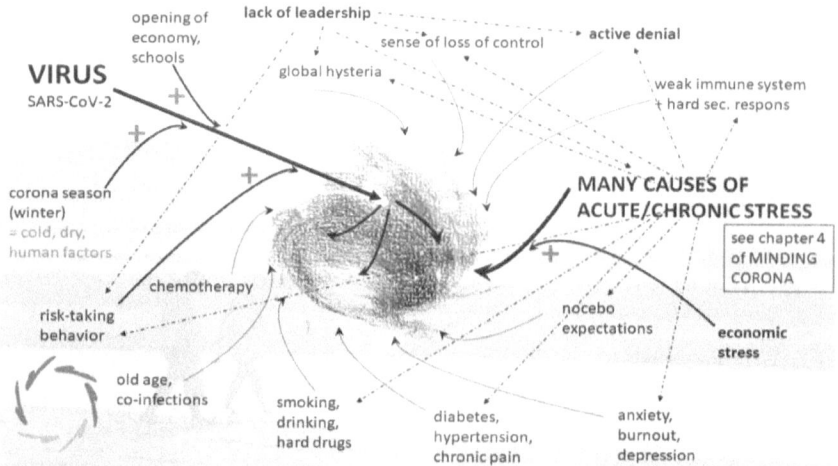

One should not think 'mind' in a dualistic setting. Body-mind unity is, by now, totally scientific. Denying this is like denying that the earth is round. Therefore, we should take the consequence at heart, urgently at present, and more widely in medicine and beyond. For instance, ironically, what used to be scientific medicine has now become unscientific if not taking into account the ton of science that has become available about the deeper mind.

As to COVID

If the bird keeps dabbling on one wing, the COVID-whirlpool will act as a turbo. I've read many times that "this virus acts in strange, incomprehensible ways." Indeed, but much of the strangeness is more related to us – our mind, our depth – than to the piece of RNA. I see in the management of COVID a huge lack of respect for who we are. Every human being is immensely more interesting and important than we care to acknowledge.

The total human species seems to keep looking right through the depth of human mind without taking notice, even in these trying times. In such case, we can foresee more COVID-deaths in the future than in the past, on top of more related disaster. Much of this can be prevented if we act right now without delay. This will be proven in a few years with the best

A.I.-driven science of that day. I'll summarize it in a postscript to my book MINDING CORONA.

This text is date-stamped and will stay so. People and organizations will forever be responsible for listening, or not listening.

As to me

Before COVID, I was busy with A.I., finishing a book The Journey Towards Compassionate A.I. This is a fascinating and worthwhile domain. It might be used – urgently – towards developing more support to us, humans, in these times of corona. Otherwise, there is a vast horizon to the ocean of A.I.

Unfortunately, Western medicine has been built on a Cartesian dualism of body and mind from which it has not yet emancipated despite all the neurocognitive science that shows the wrongness of this basic premise. This has many dire consequences concerning many health-related issues. One of them is the way we are handling the present-day calamity. It is mind-boggling that every physician can delve into this domain and see the implications for medicine. It's still not happening, yet the tension is growing. We cannot go on like this. At least, my published writings are and will remain a sad legacy.

Anyway, don't wait for me on the COVID trail. We can only do this together. Dear reader, you give this bird a second wing, and it will fly.

The alternative is a human-made disaster on top of the viral accident.

Yep, it's also emotional. Among other things, what happens at the other side of the world at present happens nearby. It's a small planet in a big universe.

Take, for instance, Argentina

"There is no economy without health." [https://www.who.int/news-room/feature-stories/detail/argentina-there-is-no-economy-without-health]

Daily New Cases in Argentina

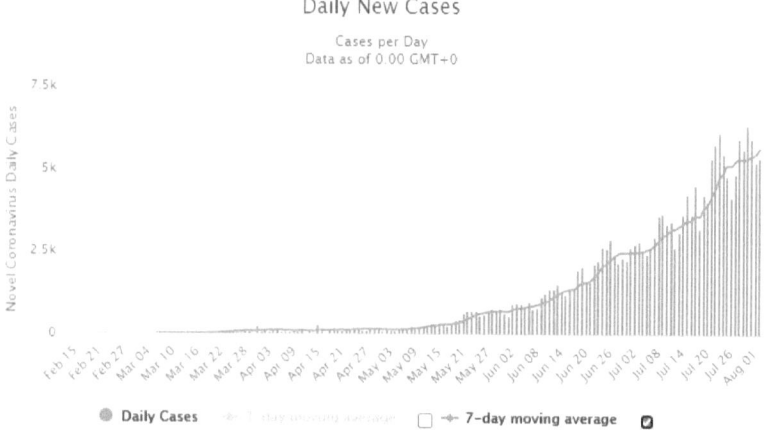

(from https://www.worldometers.info/)

Deaths are also surging now. What is happening here?

Argentina went into an early and severe lockdown. Argentina's President Alberto Fernández argued this, saying: "You can recover from a drop in the GDP, but you can't recover from death." That's the most humane thing to do, absolutely!

But the economy is falling through the bottom. The country is opening because there is no choice. Already in recession before the pandemic, a projected 7.3% contraction in GDP predicts 45% of the population living in poverty.

Note that it is wintertime in the southern hemisphere. Nevertheless, temperatures in Buenos Aires are like the spring in Belgium (8-18°C). Thus, there is no disproof of corona seasonality at all in this, nor in any other known fact. One can confidently predict two things:

- From the middle of September onwards, Argentina will fare better as to COVID (not the economy).

- In Europe and the US, a few weeks later, the real ordeal only starts.

I can't help it. My heart is bleeding from all this.

23. The Final COVID Question: Ethics or Economics?

August 4, 2020

	Today	Total
Cases worldwide	**254,988**	**18,692,376**
Deaths worldwide	**6,298**	**703,381**

Putting ethics and economics against each other indicates that in this question, I see economics as non-ethical, and ethics as non-economical.

As if that would be possible

Non-ethical would be the hallmark of a sociopath; non-economical that of either an utterly naïve person or a Buddhist at the brink of parinirvana.

In normal society, there is always an intermingling. Putting ethics and economics purely against each other is stuff for a thought experiment. Such can teach us something without necessarily being possible, except as a thought. Nevertheless, it can clarify choices.

Health or money?

This is the more frequently asked question, but to me, in many cases, 'health' is used implicitly to point to, eventually, the wellbeing and even life of vulnerable people who, most frequently, are not allowed to choose in this. Implicitly, it's the strong-and-healthy who decide. For instance, older people just undergo.

On top of this, implicit is also, in many cases, that the rich choose for the poor. Opting for the money is choosing against those without it. So, in this choice, frequently and implicitly, money is not put in the balance with health, but with no-money. Even more clearly put: the powerful versus the non-powerful.

Hmm. Making it explicit doesn't make it easier to swallow, does it? One can still discuss the meanings of terms, but at least, it's more open to avoid implicit assumptions if possible.

So, I prefer the question: ethics or economics?

Ethics may be seen very broadly. It's about the vulnerable in homes for the elderly. It's also about immensely lonely adolescents, maltreated wives and husbands, individuals who cannot afford a million USD in hospitalization costs in NYC, refugees in Bangladesh, and starving kids in Africa.

It's about all this, and how we deal with all this. The most unethical stance would be to not care for any of them, not even to want to think about them, to run away to some moral desert, sticking one's head in the sand of which there's enough.

At least, we can suffer for those who suffer. From that suffering – the former one – we can take a better look upon what to do. Maybe, with little effort, one can do much? Not asking this question doesn't lead to a valid answer.

There is no judgment in the answer if it's an answer to the valid question. Each person can try to get to a personal reply, which should be respected. Maybe, someone doesn't go on vacation and gives (part of) his holiday money to a rationally good cause instead. Yeowch. Is that necessarily bad for the economy? Maybe, another person cares for the children first and saves the money. Maybe someone thinks "It's now or never" and spends lavishly. Anything is better than not posing the question itself, in-depth, profoundly. The superficial question is, of course, not a question but a bunch of meaningless syllables.

The question will become very important indeed.

It has already been pertinent in this pandemic. It will increasingly become so with each next wave. We may as well get used to it. This virus is here to stay. In the third and probably also the fourth world, the additional misery from it will linger on for years.

As in wartime, some get richer; most get poorer. It becomes increasingly harder not to make the first choice. And to a substantial degree, it is a choice, not just a coincidence.

The kids! The kids! And the grandchildren! Yes, indeed. It's part of being human to have to make such choices. So, what is the most ethical choice? You see, that's why an easy judgment is inappropriate. There is no guilt in making any choice. There is, in my view, much responsibility in going deep inside to find the answer to a question that stays relevant for a lifetime.

Did I make the right choice(s) in these times of COVID? If I wouldn't bother about it, I didn't. If it wouldn't keep me awake at night sometimes even after years, I didn't.

The question is also immensely interesting.

This is mainly because it invites one to grow as a person. In this sense, COVID can be an excellent teacher. I explicitly and with much emphasis say 'can.' One has to be open to this teacher. One has to earn the teaching. This teacher doesn't teach for nothing.

"And what's in it for me," one may ask, "in this 'growing' that you talk about?" "Well," I may respond, "the answer to this specific question will be the result of your growing."

And I add, I repeat, that it's immensely interesting.

Argentina

Remember from a previous text: "You can recover from a drop in the GDP, but you can't recover from death." This is a choice for ethics, whatever comes after it (and the Argentinians too are not at the end of it). Maybe it's a proper idea to go to Buenos Aires after all this, peso-less but dancing the tango day and night with an unstained soul.

Ah, tango, the dance that teaches to be present in the present. One can linger in solitude and yet be as close as possible to another person in body and mind (and soul). In times of COVID and social distancing, also frequently in body and mind (and soul), being in the present in togetherness – even with the kid in Bangladesh – is what makes us worthy human beings. Maybe, in this setting, we are allowed to stay on this planet for a while longer.

Ethics or economics?

The question becomes really interesting when looking for answers that form a synthesis of ethics and economics — doing well by doing good. It enables one to do even better by doing better. Sounds attractive.

Indeed, but it presupposes much hard work, creativity, asking and answering real questions from really deep, not being content before one has turned oneself inside out. Never giving up. Choosing, in business – whether profit or non-profit – for sustainability, humility, solidarity, and tenacity. No fear of being contrarian.

Thus, a choice for economics for the sake of ethics. An inclusive society includes the non-powerful. A Compassionate society takes care of the non-powerful.

This is not naïve. This is real.

It's also a set of immensely difficult choices nowadays. If we feel it this way, then we are a good species. If the COVID pandemic could help us in this, then it's a worthwhile, excruciatingly awful accident.

24. COVID + School + Children

August 16, 2020

	Today	Total
Cases worldwide	**284.357**	**21.058.148**
Deaths worldwide	**6.649**	**756.719**

Corona: just a kind of flu?

In a way, and even after all that has happened and before all that will happen still, it is probably correct. Look at Southeast Asia. Even in the democratic West, if conceptually *and* subconceptually, we would have done the right things from the start on, or even from now on, the virus wouldn't dictate us as it does by far. Would the misery be little, as in flu-like? Nobody knows. But I dare say: probably. Even from now on, the pain (the deaths, the wounded, the financially devastated) would diminish drastically.

A few years from now, A.I.-driven real-world evidence may show whether or not this is correct.

Schools will reopen in Europe and the US.

At least a large number of them. Way too many and too open. After weeks, the situation will be unbearable. Will this be mainly school-driven? Nobody will 'know for sure.'

Yet this will cause a surplus of many deaths and other mishaps for sure.

Due to pressure, schools should again be partially closed.

So far, so obvious. That's why I don't question it. I assert it.

Did 'the virus' surprise you? It has negatively surprised me several times already. Time and again, I see mayhem coming, but I'm surprised by how quickly. Of course, if you reckon with a COVID-whirlpool, you don't know how strong the current is if you're not inside.

So, I give the school re-closing ample time. Six to eight weeks? I may be wrong again. I would so much like to be wrong positively!

Of course, everybody wants to do good for the children.

And their parents. And the economy for which the parents need to work instead of educating their children.

And the economists who see that we financially don't survive the second lockdown in the way of the first one. We're still unsure whether we'll financially survive the first one. Many individuals and small companies will not. Yet the general population is hardly aware of

> second lockdown → probable meltdown → socio-economic-political whirlpool

I am getting nervous

'For the good of the children' is not good for the children. Unfortunately, the children will suffer in any case. By rashly opening schools, all in all, they will suffer more, not less.

Apart from hard economics, I see short-sighted empathy — or call it *sympathy* in this respect [see: "Landscape of Empathy"] — as a human asset that doesn't always serve us well. This kind of empathy/sympathy may make one think that "at least, my small-part-of-the-world will not fare worse than the adjacent parts." That is probably correct. What one does on top of this is an ethical choice with everlasting consequence.

Of course, everybody wants to do good for 'the children.' And in the first stage, it will be good for 'the children.' One can also distribute an infinite number of cigarettes for free. In the first stage, it will be good for smokers. But?

But?

> Only a small amount of children got positive tests in the spring.

>< The kids didn't go to school, nor their teachers. It was spring, not the runny-nose season of autumn, nor the full corona-season of winter. Teachers had time and energy to be extremely cautious. 'Motivation fatigue' is not so much scientific as it is real. Also, kids may have negative tests while being infectious.

> Contact tracing didn't point much to children during the last few months.

>< Children may be test-negative yet infect each other, such as by sticking mutual objects in their mouths, by frequently hugging each other, by not taking care in which direction they cough. -> It's tough to contact-trace. With many people infected, there are always others who seem suspect besides the children. Also, children might infect adults while not getting sick. Then the adult may get ill and spread more virus to the child who then tests positive. This can be seen as an adult → child infection while it is the reverse.

OK. Don't put too much effort in the right-or-wrong of this. The spring is not the autumn. My point is that nothing is straightforward. We need to live with uncertainties, following science as well as we can.

Science (at least some, by now) about children and schools

I did my homework. A few top-notch scientific studies are revealing.

Ludvigsson, in a systematic review, points out that "Children are unlikely to be the main drivers of the pandemic. **Opening up schools and kindergartens is unlikely to impact COVID-19 mortality rates in older** people." [Ludvigsson, 2020] **Unfortunately, this study doesn't distinguish between the ages of children. It appears to be concerning the little ones.** Also, many of the studies in the review are small and seem flawed. Still, it's a worthwhile study in general terms.

A German study finds **viral loads to be less, but still quite substantial in symptomatic children versus symptomatic adults.** Small symptomatic children (0-10 years) have less viral loads than the 11-20 years group. [Jones et al., 2020]

An excellent study from South Korea, yet to be published (but already accepted) identified 5,706 people who were the first to report Covid-19 symptoms in their households between January 20 and March 27, when schools were closed, tracing the 59,073 contacts of these "index cases." This study shows that **older <u>infected</u> children (10-19 years) spread SARS-CoV-2 as much if not more than adults, while younger children do so much less although still substantially: around half that of all other ages together.** [Park et al., 2020] I find 'half' very much! A limitation of the study, acknowledged by the researchers: the first person in a household to develop symptoms is not necessarily the first to have been infected. This way, the study may have <u>under</u>estimated the number of children who set off the chain of transmission within their households. The study also doesn't show how efficiently non-symptomatic children spread the virus.

An article in *Science* about Chinese experiences concludes that (with bold by me) "Although proactive school closures cannot interrupt transmission on their own, they **can reduce peak incidence by 40 to 60% and delay the epidemic.**" [Zhang et al., 2020] This and other research in Argentina, Italy and South Korea [Neidhofer et al., 2020] shows that school-closure needs to be done early and drastically in order to have this optimum effect.

On July 30, a *Lancet* article concludes, very sensibly (with highlight by me): "To prevent a second COVID-19 wave, relaxation of physical distancing, including reopening of schools, in the UK **must be accompanied by large-scale, population-wide testing of symptomatic**

individuals and effective tracing of their contacts, followed by isolation of diagnosed individuals." [Panovska-Griffiths et al., 2020] Otherwise, and together with reopening of society, they warn of "a resulting second wave of infections 2.0 – 2.3 times the size of the original COVID-19 wave." They also see a second wave peak in December 2020 versus February 2021. As I understand this, it's twice as long, twice as hard. That makes four. It's just numbers, but in my view, with COVID-whirlpool-turbo on top, this is not an underestimate. Let us be extraordinarily cautious and SLOW.

My take on this: small children are, fortunately, no killer-bombs. COVID-adolescents are as infective as adults. But they get COVID-ill in smaller (although apparently already mounting in time) numbers. On the other hand, they may get common colds in higher numbers, spreading SARS-CoV-2 virus this way. Also, one should look at direct contacts *and* at second-degree contacts *and* so on. Top-notch contact tracing is indeed a must. Without it, opening schools is a behind-the-screen cause of many deaths. Without it, one cannot choose for the former without the latter.

An non-exhaustive enumeration of what may furthermore go wrong.

[Note the COVID-whirlpool [see: "COVID-Whirlpool"] in every following point, without mentioning it.]

- When a teenager is the size of an adult, he is equally infective. He is, pragmatically seen, even more infective than an adult. He is an unknown spreader for a substantial amount of days. Also, teenagers may have 'unhygienic habits.' No guilt to them, of course. It's just what it is. This condition is related to uneven brain development (amygdalae versus prefrontal cortex, up to 23 years of   age). [https://www.aacap.org/AACAP/Families_and_Youth/Facts_for_Families/FFF-Guide/The-Teen-Brain-Behavior-Problem-Solving-and-Decision-Making-095.aspx]

- School teachers are going to get sick. Some will die. Others will quit. Replacements will not be easy to find.

- Also, partners will get COVID or be anxious about getting it. They may not want to cohabit with their possible death sentence.

- Healthcare workers get school-COVID patients, of whom they know that the risks have been taken with more or less conscious intent. This will be emotionally extra hard.

- Teachers and students will be seen as guilty of school-borne infections, not taking precautions well enough. A number of them will indeed do so and be found guilty by others.

- Parents' parents will die. Increasingly, it will become apparent, also through tracing, that a substantial source is school-bound. By then, too late for many. Lifelong, children-of-now will know they 'caused' their grandparents dying.

- After a while, parents will make this deduction by themselves, and it will be in social and other media.

- Symptoms from a common cold and flu will get much attention, provoking much anxiety.

- The sensitivity and specificity of COVID tests will show its (low-level) worth in these specific circumstances of high prevalence and vague symptoms. This adds to people's losing confidence in experts and expertise, making non-science flourish.

- We are giving the virus ample resources to learn to adapt to children -> detrimental mutations in the make. This is already going on. It's a logical move by the virus, seeking broader habitats in the same way as it founds humans in 2019. It cannot help it. That's what a virus does. However, this particular virus is more dangerous in this respect than most others.

- What with the safety of mentally disabled children and their teachers?

Back to the whirlpool. I don't see this being taken into account anywhere. The situation with versus without whirlpool is comparable to a linear versus logarithmic progression. Or, if you like, something like a summation versus a multiplication in which, additionally, the terms themselves get bigger.

In a schema, with t for time and d for disaster:

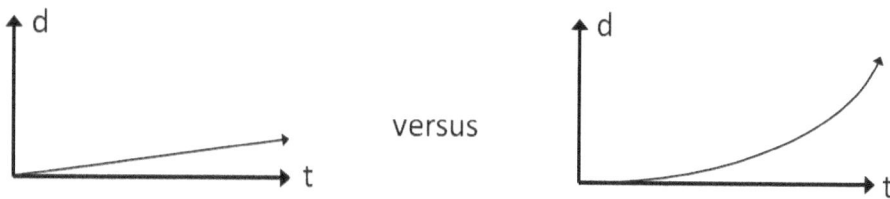

Bye, bye, control. I wish you were here.

"But we didn't see this coming!"

"Then, you didn't read MINDING CORONA!" On top of that, you didn't read the scientific literature very well. Dear reader, this makes me immensely sad. Please don't throw any guilt to anyone. It's not worth it, and it's counterproductive.

But do let us be sad together.

We're entitled to be so.

I wonder whether politicians are betting on a timely miracle cure (will not happen) and are willing to ram through a huge surplus number of deaths and wounded (complications) to 'save the economy.' Is the plan, for the sake of money, to accept a second wave four times as hard as the first one? Dearest reader, would it be acceptable to you? If in any country or part of the world, politicians have this plan, then I can tell them: You don't know what you are meddling with. You see one part of the picture, and it may well be the smallest part. Your plan to 'save the economy' may thus backfire into even more economic ship-wrecking.

Some countries have successfully reopened schools, while others have closed them down again. The number of community cases to close down schools varies wildly from country to country. For instance, South Korea, despite very good contact-tracing in place, closed down 840 schools based on some 80 new cases (not deaths) on one day. [https://www.businessinsider.nl/hundreds-south-korean-schools-

closed-amid-spike-coronavirus-cases-2020-5?international=true&r=US]
Belgium had 922 cases yesterday, with – everybody agrees – suboptimal contact-tracing in place.

Any alternative for schooling?

That is: apart from my theoretical and practical developments. The app! The app! My kingdom for the app! And it's for free! And it's apparently... for another planet.

One doesn't need to be a pedagogue to see that for the kids, challenging times are unavoidable. Since school is impossible, and no-school is impossible, one needs to jump out of the box and into another box. Let's try one. I call this 'micro-schooling.'

Micro-schooling

The main idea is simple. Call me naïve if you like, but for some of you, my readers, the direction has crossed your mind already. Your further intelligence is needed to make an elephant into a mosquito.

It's not applicable for all children, but for most, probably, at least with some additional insights in 'deep motivation,' etc. Also, this is not new. From country to country, already, aspects of this are being promoted or realized.

The basic idea: put four children together, let them be responsible for each other to quite some degree. Every four to six weeks, groups may change. Let all group members be accountable individually and for each other within that group. Of course, they should have the means to communicate with each other. Computer? Coming together at school now and then: four children in one classroom along with a teacher?

What's in it for each?

- For the teacher, micro-school-bubbles are more workable than contacting every pupil individually.
- For the students, they learn invaluable lessons in co-creation, co-responsibility, co-motivation, even leadership.

- For the parents who are willing and able to do so: let the micro-schools (four children) be together during the day in one house, with one parent. Three others can go to work.
- For society: economy can hopefully keep going.

Just an idea. More important: the circumstance obliges us to be super-out-of-the-box-thinking.

That needs openness and respect.

And above all, it needs us to discover who we are and why it matters.

References

[Zhang et al., 2020] Zhang J, Litvinova M, Liang Y, et al. Changes in contact patterns shape the dynamics of the COVID-19 outbreak in China. *Science*. 2020;368(6498):1481-1486. doi:10.1126/science.abb8001

[Neidhofer et al., 2020] The Effectiveness of School Closures and Other Pre-Lockdown COVID-19 Mitigation Strategies in Argentina, Italy, and South Korea --- Claudio Neidhofer, Guido Neidhofer - This version: July 3, 2020

[Ludvigsson, 2020] Ludvigsson JF. Children are unlikely to be the main drivers of the COVID-19 pandemic - A systematic review. *Acta Paediatr*. 2020;109(8):1525-1530. doi:10.1111/apa.15371

[Panovska-Griffiths et al., 2020] Panovska-Griffiths J, Kerr CC, Stuart RM, et al. Determining the optimal strategy for reopening schools, the impact of test and trace interventions, and the risk of occurrence of a second COVID-19 epidemic wave in the UK: a modelling study [published online ahead of print, 2020 Aug 3]. *Lancet Child Adolesc Health*. 2020;S2352-4642(20)30250-9. doi:10.1016/S2352-4642(20)30250-9

[Park et al., 2020] https://wwwnc.cdc.gov/eid/article/26/10/20-1315 article Park YJ, Choe YJ, Park O, et al. Contact Tracing during Coronavirus Disease Outbreak, South Korea, 2020 [published online ahead of print, 2020 Jul 16]. *Emerg Infect Dis.* 2020;26(10):10.3201/eid2610.201315. doi:10.3201/eid2610.201315

[Jones et al., 2020] Jones TC, Mühlemann B, Veith T, et al. An analysis of SARS-CoV-2 viral load by patient age (https://zoonosen.charite.de/fileadmin/user_upload/microsites/m_cc05/virologieccm/ dateien_upload/Weitere_Dateien/analysis-of-SARS-CoV-2-viral-load-by-patient-age.pdf). German Research network Zoonotic Infectious Diseases website: Charité - Universitätsmedizin Berlin, 2020.

25. COVID
Compassion

August 19, 2020

	Today	Total
Cases worldwide	272.021	22.569.598
Deaths worldwide	6.668	790.190

Compassion is not 'empathy.'

Apart from terminological issues [see: "Landscape of Empathy"], empathy can be narrow or broad. Empathy for only-the-own-bubble may thwart broad empathy. This way, it may be a source of us-versus-them feelings: 'Us' needs protection against 'them, the enemy.'

On feelings of anxiety and frustration, such empathy may evolve towards aggression. That is not Compassion. It may also lead to an increasing short-sightedness, like 'sticking one's head in the sand' until one's head is lost, possibly including that of some other(s) in the small bubble. That is also not Compassion. Please, don't make such a mistake.

Neither is Compassion opposed to empathy. Empathy is a necessary but insufficient characteristic of Compassion. Sorry for the theory. Some more will pass in order to understand the present situation.

The present situation

is one in which Compassion is central. Compassion looks at deaths and other tolls not only as numbers. Worldwide, far-reaching and necessary decisions profoundly depend on this. Actually, they always do, but it happens more openly now and with starkly direct consequences for different groups. The following are a few examples.

The elderly

are specifically vulnerable to the disease and to head-on loneliness. On top of that, to the dying in solitude, quarantined one way or another.

Also, according to studies, more than 90% of deaths are people > 65 years of age. Thus, COVID-19 is sometimes described as a 'disease of the elderly' as if it's, therefore, less important.

They need our Compassion.

Youth

have other vulnerabilities, not so much to the disease, but to being kept from their peers, and to experiencing difficulties in social, mental, and educational development. On top of that, they cannot readily talk about it face-to-face.

Also, they will pay for the expenses being made to 'save the economy.' With a continuing pandemic, they may do so for a very long time.

They need our Compassion.

Those suffering economically

Losing one's income, seeing one's lifework going down or even down the drain, losing one's home, one's self-worth, one's dreams, one's sense of being responsible, and 'doing the proper thing.' This multifaceted suffering is diverse and different in different parts of the world.

It can make a broader kind of empathy difficult. Generally, stress makes one's empathic vision narrower. In collective and tremendous stress, with borders of the discomfort zone getting nearer, frustrations may mount.

They need our Compassion.

But what's in it to say that "we just have to live with the virus" as if that's a fact? That would be the most terrible, inhuman mistake!

"But for the sake of the economy, we need to…" But for the sake of <u>what</u> would we need such an economy? Please enlighten me with something meaningful, something deeper than the tapestry on the wall. Without a wall, the tapestry is just a miserable heap of wrinkled paper.

Increasingly

We are heading towards a coronated autumn and winter. Several factors make the situation worse. People are more vulnerable than before through psychological and economic hurt. Additionally, the virus will hit harder in its preferred season – winter – in Europe and the US.

Unfortunately, people didn't miraculously become more Compassionate in the last few months. On the contrary, they have become less patient, more fed-up and burned-out, more stressed generally. There is seemingly less Compassion around. That's bad for the immune system and for how people behave socially.

In my view, we need Compassion more than ever.

Compassion, not an easy concept!

The capital 'C' denotes that the subconceptual level is intrinsic to Compassion. It is also essential to human intelligence and consciousness. With 'subconceptual' [see: "About 'Subconceptual'"], I indicate +/- nonconscious mental, meaningful processing as it is being uncovered through highest-level scientific research in the cognitive neuroscience domain. In my book *Your Mind as Cure*, I show that insight into this level is necessary to understand how we can get ill through the mind and cured through the mind.

Rationality consists of reckoning with the conceptual as well as the subconceptual level. Taking into account only one of them is unscientific. To understand Compassion, we also need both. There is no Compassion without at least a substantial openness towards rationality.

Not egoism, nor altruism.

Compassion transcends both. It may make one 'feel good' when doing good for someone else. That is not being foolish. It is about being ethical. It's self-orientedness without losing sight of the other, and other-orientedness without losing sight of oneself. This may be understood mainly at the conceptual level while being realized at the subconceptual level.

No more theory, I promise → back to COVID.

Why we need COVID Compassion

We cannot leave any people behind. As said, my list of three groups is meant as a working tool. One might also see different races, sexes, classes, parts of the world, subcultures, religions. The principles of Compassion are always the same. Eventually, there is only one group involved in COVID: the human group (and some bats). But without Compassion, people will not continue abiding by the rules. One can see ample examples of this already.

We need Compassion because it's ethical as well as the most efficient way. Without Compassion, we need rules to make sure that different groups don't turn against each other.

We need to take care of retired people, working people, and youth, even if it doesn't appear to be possible. Many measures have to be taken for the good of one group that are apparently bad for another. Think of lockdown. In competition, any measure can engender resistance. Imposing rules is an element within this competition. Face masks or no face masks? Who gets the power to impose the rules and coerce others to follow them? Who will abandon these rules *en masse*? Who already knows they will do so? Do you call that efficient?!

Not me.

First Compassion, then rules

In other words: true leadership. This doesn't mean that rules are less important. It implies that Compassion is crucial. Compassion comes first. It may be thought of without rules. Rules may not, in any sensible way, be thought of without Compassion.

Thus, if one brings rules in sensitive COVID situations, it should be done from a basis of Compassion. Not rules as being about the rules themselves, or out of 'being the expert' as if that is ever enough. We all need to be experts in being human. In every discussion and communication about why some rule is required, Compassion should be deeply present. Otherwise, as we see time and again, the communication may eventually be counter-productive.

COVID, this way, can become a daily exercise in Compassion. This may be the only way to keep going. It motivates. It makes people stronger to continue abiding by the rules. It makes people less anxious, less stressed, thus also better personally equipped to overcome the virus itself.

Not simple

One might think this is just a thing to do. Contrary to this, Compassion is a challenging process of growth. It's never finished. Every Compassionate experience may add to it, like a mature art that still continuously gets better. As said, this is why true leadership is crucial and may save many lives. True leadership is Compassionate. A true leader is always growing into this kind of leadership.

When one thinks there's a short way, there's certainly a long way ahead.

Compassion and mental aftermath

We already see much mental suffering, of which much is not officially recognized at present. There will undoubtedly be more loneliness, guilt, mourning, anxiety, loneliness again, depression. Stress of all sorts.

Compassion brings people profoundly together. It also brings one closer to oneself, leading to inner strength and resilience. It leads to inner growth. It starts from who one is and can become, whether young, middle-aged, or old. Mental distress doesn't come so much from circumstances as from interpretations of the circumstances. How they are remembered; how they are integrated or precisely not into broader schemes that one builds up as meaningful mental landscapes in which to explore a full life. Compassion has a huge influence on such interpretations, personally and interpersonally. Compassion makes them deeper and stronger, more open, more respectful.

Without this, one can get genuinely lonely and distressed.

Much suffering can be alleviated

through Compassion not as the source of action but as the action itself: the feeling Compassion, the being Compassionate.

This doesn't mean that bread is simply unimportant. Without bread, one dies. But without poetry — the poetic or 'subconceptual' or Compassionate side of the human being — one is dead already. We should take care of both.

This way, the different needs of different groups can be met in-depth, even if it seems impossible if one looks only at the surface. People are not mere surfaces. They are, always and everywhere, complete human beings. They need to be seen as such. This may be wondrous, even incomprehensible, if looked at from the surface, yet the most profound need of any human being is to be seen in totality. A ton of superficial attention is not worth one gram of deep attention. Another word for the latter is Compassion.

This insight is becoming more and more urgently needed.

26. MINDING CORONA, Saving Livelihoods and Lives

August 22, 2020

	Today	Total
Cases worldwide	258.252	23.108.416
Deaths worldwide	6.062	802.600

The causal role of the mind on COVID is being given the cold shoulder, not therefore consciously, but effectively indeed. It doesn't 'culturally fit.'

WHAT – A – PITY

The result is unnecessary deaths and economic downfall, causing more human misery.

It may also be the death of your business or loved one(s). I guess that's important. Yet many people who – should – know better keep quiet. They go with the flow.

Why?

Apparently, to them, it's <u>not</u> that important after all?

This text is addressed to those who can easily make a difference, who think themselves rational, but many aren't from the moment it's personally challenging. Indeed, it may make one a cultural misfit.

Where are the brave?

Hiding the mind as a causal factor is starkly UNscientific at present. As the relevant science progresses, this is more and more the case in many fields of healthcare. As has happened many times in the past, part of yesterday's 'regular medicine' is becoming tomorrow's quackery.

Yet I hear it many times, by people about others and themselves. It concerns media people, scientists, politicians, influencers:

People don't dare to talk about the mind as a causal factor in COVID.

This way, the virus gets quite a free rein during the next year in the developed world, much longer elsewhere.

We know increasingly more about the disease and, fortunately, about how to manage it. Also, we 'know' there will be no miracle vaccine, just as there is still none for influenza (*). Also, there is no miracle cure in sight. The one that was most promising in my view – convalescent plasma therapy – was put on hold by the FDA a few days ago after months of intense enthusiasm from scientists and despite an ongoing controversy, now citing weak data (placebo related) from the most extensive study to date. This is the best way to perform science. It shows how challenging science can be.

[Note, by the way, my placebo related critiques of remdesivir [see my book MINDING CORONA]. Concerning plasma, the FDA just saved me from writing another letter to the editor of the New England Journal of Medicine.]

Of course, we don't know the future, but come on, be serious.

Also, we know what people should do to avoid contagion, and we know they will not, or, in large parts of the world, cannot. We also know much of the why on both occasions.

That leaves us with our mind as the most promising cure

(to be investigated with utmost urgency if you please. A free app is at your disposal.)

But then why is the mind hardly mentioned as such? The way this has been going on for half a year is mind-boggling. The mind, seriously, even in potential, as a causal factor in COVID, is nowhere in science. Also, hardly in popular media.

Readers of MINDING CORONA can see that my thinking went to the mind in March 2020, with sadness, at a global death count of 9.000. There is much science from different directions backing this. I'm not complaining, just pointing out what may well become, in retrospect, the consequence of a maddening situation, date-stamped, open to anyone.

This book isn't finished. Globally, we're at 800.000 deaths, officially. That makes at least 1.2 million in reality if you know anything about this world. My worst-case was 3 million. Now I see we are going to soar right beyond that. Still, the deep mind may remain invisible. Unfathomable.

Contacts and some loneliness

I contacted people who I thought would be interested. There was some interest, indeed, in the sense of "You might well be correct, but shut your mouth; this is not the time to come forward with such. It's too dangerous." Or, one after the other: "There is no time, no occasion. I don't want to. Just leave me alone. I'm on vacation. I will contact you (nope)."

Some of my friends, as the saying goes, disappeared, becoming untouchable.

Indeed, that feels lonely. I know now.

No fearmongering, please!

There's a big difference between fearmongering and telling people facts (even fuzzy ones) about what is bound to happen. I regularly pose someone the question about how they would organize life in two near-future alternatives: COVID-disaster or COVID-blue-sky. Many would act VERY differently. That's important because the COVID-whirlpool will (again) make a huge difference, with a big role for the mind. [see: "Only 'Control' + COVID-Whirlpool = DISASTER"] This is not a game.

Telling people a fact-based opinion is rational, challenging, and Compassionate. [see: "COVID Compassion"] Throwing people (again) in a whirlpool without every possible substantial measure of defense is not Compassionate. It may look friendlier. But when the time comes and people get into panic mode, it's too late.

Also, look at the world situation, with arguably 10.000 deaths per day. True, this is a small part of daily mortality. True, there are other infectious diseases with a high death toll. But that is no <u>excuse</u> for these deaths. In my view, there is no <u>excuse</u> for even one single premature preventable death. What about you?

The main lesson is about deep mind.

This is really invisible in present-day medicine. I had no idea that this is so, well, almost total. Or what? There's much anxiety in this regard. As to COVID, everybody seems to wait for everybody. Even so, one loud voice and the heads disappear even deeper into the desert sand. I would gladly take any challenge. Meanwhile, COVID reigns

and keeps reigning

and keeps reigning.

Ironically, the sector that is supposed to teach us about human depth, the cultural sector, is largely being ignored for the sake of the economy. No money for depth. Isn't that precisely an essential cause of the happening?

Will the real mind eventually come forward?

Science progresses rapidly. That's why it is so valuable; not because it's immutable, but precisely because it's mutable. Especially in the last few years, scientific developments are promising. These go from unexpectedly in-depth visualization of nerve patterns in the brain, to artificial intelligence techniques for discerning patterns in the human mind with a potentially huge influence on health, and to a growing emphasis in medical science on real-world data and pragmatic trials. Thus, we are seeing the dawn of a new, additional kind of health-related science: no extrapolations from randomized controlled trials, but real-world evidence driven by Artificial Intelligence. This will show which mind-related factors make people ill and better again.

There may be more already, hidden in labs or scientific journals, like viruses ready to leap to mainstream. Post-corona, it will show relatively soon what we could have done but didn't. In retrospect, it will be unimaginable that this could happen in 2020.

In 2020!

Who will dare to say in 2030. "I didn't see this obvious thing?" Or even in 2025? Or even in 2022 if I get what I want in time?

I keep on writing MINDING CORONA.

So tired of this virus.

One cannot escape it. I mean, the talk about it. And rest assured, my wife is even more tired of it than you are since I have been intensely writing this book. I wish the thing would miraculously disappear.

Imagine I'm right. In that case, I may be given the Nobel prize and give it directly to research.

Imagine. Then how many people could have been helped profoundly? We're talking millions. If I don't get through the mindless veil, it will not be done. This is the weirdest situation.

At least study it.

If the mind were a pill with similar indications of efficacy, billions would flow to its use in prevention and management. Nothing flows to it now except the little that I can spend on it, making an app that can change the course of the world if the world cares to listen.

For many years, I have been delving into the science of mind-body-unity and the influence of mind on the body. I compare medical science to an ivory tower with an unscientific swamp on all sides. Since mind-body-unity doesn't get a proper place in the tower, it's drowned in the swamp.

WHAT – A – PITY

The deeply meaningful mind has been denigrated for millennia.

It's high time we wake up to it.

Meanwhile, to 'go with the flow' is not rational by definition. 'The flow' is not a rational argument. It has never been one. Even more, Western Enlightenment, one of our primary sources of pride, has come into existence out of a desire to <u>not</u> go with the flow in science and rationality. Therefore, it's especially unfortunate to see it happen so gratuitously in the matter of COVID.

I write this to an open future, hopefully, a very near one.

(*) Science is not always easy, especially for scientists with an ego. Interesting in this regard is the Cochrane report from 2018: "Vaccines for preventing influenza in the elderly" (https://doi.org/10.1002/14651858.CD004876.pub4). *Cochrane* is like scientific heaven. They work with the utmost rigor. In this case, they searched all highest-level medical, scientific databases for evidence (Randomized Controlled Trials) from 1966 till 2017. Some quotes from their report with highlights by me:

- "Older adults receiving the influenza vaccine may have a lower risk of Influenza (from 6% to 2.4%)… These results indicate that **30 people would need to be vaccinated to prevent one person experiencing influenza.**"
- "The evidence for a lower risk of Influenza and ILI with vaccination is **limited by biases in the design or conduct of the studies. Lack of detail regarding the methods used to confirm the diagnosis of influenza limits the applicability of this result.** The available evidence relating to complications is of poor quality, insufficient, or old and provides no clear guidance for public health regarding the safety, efficacy, or effectiveness of influenza vaccines for people aged 65 years or older. Society

should invest in research on a new generation of influenza vaccines for the elderly."

- "The study providing data for mortality and pneumonia was underpowered to detect differences in these outcomes. There were 3 deaths from 522 participants in the vaccination arm and 1 death from 177 participants in the placebo arm, providing **very low-certainty evidence for the effect on mortality**."

So apparently, this is the conclusion in the case of influenza from the beacon of science after decades of investigation: arguably 3% less chance of getting the disease; 0% less chance of dying from it. That might seem a bit weird to someone who doesn't appreciate the importance of prevalence in statistics. Also, there is poor quality evidence about safety. Of course, other vaccines, such as those against measles and polio, are super life-savers. Is COVID more like polio or more like influenza? The general scientific agreement points to the latter.

27. The Problem with Corona is the Problem with Medicine

September 16, 2020

	Daily	Total
Cases worldwide	308.870	30.027.119
Deaths worldwide	6.224	944.715

I mean, in anything mind-related. This is not about the body-as-pure-body.
►►►WHY read this? The mind-problem is present in the whole of medicine. Not in some subspecialty, but in all of them. ◄◄◄

Is this even possible?

Good question. In principle, it's only possible with something that lies at the basis of the whole building – like an inverted pyramid.

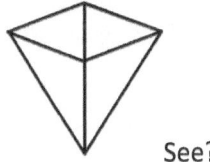 See?

At the basis lies, as I wrote in *Minding COVID, a different story*, a dual assumption that can best be grasped in synthesis. [see: "Minding COVID: a Different Story"] It's 'the tip of the pyramid' – where mind and body are most readily seen as one. Recapitulating the dual assumption:

- Mind and body are one.
- Non-conscious processing exists in meaningful ways.

If we have this wrong, we have everything wrong.

Unfortunately, we do have this wrong.

Do this simple test:

> Ask any physician where the mind is. Which answer do you expect? On a cloud? With God? In another dimension? In the brain?

OK. This is a tricky question. Every movement of the mind is a movement of the body. There is no one without the other in either direction. Let's redo the test:

> You can leave out 'soul.' Ask this same physician whether the mind can move – as while thinking about this text – without any movement of the body (the brain, at least) even at the smallest level. Which answer do you expect?

If it's 'no,' then we're pretty deep into the game of body-mind-unity. There is no influence of one on the other because it's the same thing, the same person. This accords with every bit of science on any domain. Also, in every human-related scientific field, it is the tip of the inverted pyramid.

If we have this wrong, we have everything wrong.

In medicine, for instance, we have this wrong, big time.

2020. A strange period. 'We' are very rational and at the same time excruciatingly irrational. Western medicine is partly very advanced, partly sliding back into the Middle Ages. The real mind, the complex one [see:

"Complex is not Complicated"] is getting less attention over the years due to technological advances that draw all attention.

Medicine has never grappled with mind-body-unity. In a bid to turn away from magic, Western scientific medicine has, from the start, made a move towards the science and philosophy of two centuries ago. A logical move back then. The high-status science was physics (therefore: 'physician'); the philosophy was Cartesian, based on the opposite of our dual assumption in both ways.

Two centuries ago, the pyramid received a base, and the base was wrong as we so pertinently, scientifically know now. Yet, two centuries onward – here and now – we still have the same pyramid and the same base. I owe you a little more explanation.

So, let's go inside the pyramid.

Sure, we know that stress can make us ill. Anxiety, depression, anger may aggravate many diseases. We also know that medication can influence the mind, in good and bad ways.

So, we 'know,' but actually, we merely act as if we knew, while we do not know in reality. We use terms like 'stress' and 'depression.' We use painkillers to kill the feeling of pain (which is the same as the pain itself). We do things to act on the body through the mind and on the mind through the body.

And that's it. Inside the pyramid, there is a place for the mind and a place for the body. In everything related to medical practice, they are different places. In two centuries, we have shuffled a bit around, but made no basic amendments. Do we need to?

Absolutely, we need to change this.

Look again at terms like 'stress' and 'depression.' They are ubiquitously used quite vaguely, by putting somewhat arbitrary elements together while excluding others. Frequently, there is a score involved or some physical parameter(s). This still shows the basic assumption:

- The mind is simple – no deeper meaning involved besides what can be consciously grasped in easy conceptual terms.
- This simplified kind-of-mind exists on top of the body, not intricately 'interwoven' in a myriad of ways. And even so.

I just called them dual, not binary. These assumptions, too, are eventually one and the same. They can only be grasped together as one. Only then can we see that delving into mind – again, twofold:

- is much more complex than simple terms can convey; therefore, it's much more difficult
- can 'influence' the body much more in-depth than is generally assumed in medicine, as it is in the whole of society

In short, it's much more difficult as well as much more effective if we grapple with the difficulties. If we don't, we end up with the dire present in many domains. [see: "Medically Unexplained Syndromes"]

This is not 'less science.'

On the contrary, it is finally coming out of Pre-Scientific Ages.

We desperately need to do so. Otherwise, we keep seeing many problems – actually, everything mind-related – getting ever more prominent. These problems will continue getting bigger until we know.

[And maybe I can find a place in this crazy world in which, as you can see in the news concerning ourselves, more and more magical thinking prevails again.]

In the meantime, "Where's the proof"?

Meaning: Where is the directly experimental science about these consequences of mind-body-unity?

Good question. Equally as good as "Where is the directly experimental proof of the opposite?"

Nowhere, really. At the moment, the score is 0:0. (*)

But no, taking into account theoretical as well as circumstantial proof, it's 2:0 in favor of mind-body-unity. In a few years, real-world-evidence may make it 3:0.

Even so, the biggest problem remains the pyramid itself in the whole of medicine.

Same problem with corona

With relatively little bodily cure in sight worldwide every day, thousands of people die who might be saved by considering mind-body-unity. Is this stark? Yes, it is! This includes many of those who die directly from COVID and those who die from indirect causes. The main indirect cause may become hunger and dislocation in countries such as India through economic disaster, fueled eventually by fear and anxiety for the disease. Note that at the time of writing, I am mainly talking about the immediate future. We can alleviate all this through proper insight into mind-body-unity.

Only, to accomplish this, the pyramid needs to be upended.

It's not happening.

Due to the weight of the pyramid, it will probably not happen soon. There is too much flowing in the same direction.

Unless, dear reader, you turn around.

Please do so for yourself; do it for everybody; do it for me.

(*) I can already hear the objection that the score is a favorable 1:0 due to a lot of proof, for instance, in the domain of mindfulness and its influence on stress and pain. Well, I may be too skeptical, but this proof doesn't satisfy me yet.

28. Motivating Crowds in Corona Times

September 26, 2020

	Today	Total
Cases worldwide	318.804	32.753.099
Deaths worldwide	5.818	992.978

A crowd is like an organism composed of organisms. If treated as a mechanism, it will not behave optimally, especially over time, especially concerning much-needed motivation.

►►►This is already crucial and will become even more important over the next six months. ◄◄◄

Does the following picture give a clear idea?

(https://www.worldometers.info/coronavirus)

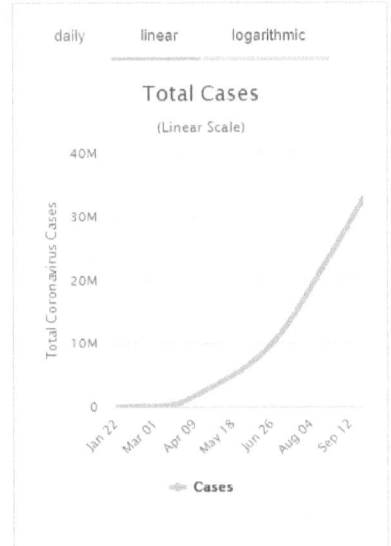

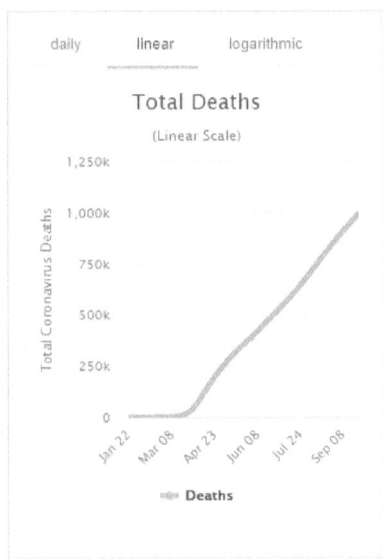

It shouldn't be this way. Living through it, I don't speak from hindsight. Maybe I don't survive next winter. Hey, perhaps you don't either. Then this text can be our witness.

In several ways, it shouldn't be this way. My specific focus – as you know by now – is subconceptual, mainly nonconscious processing, of which you can find much in my blogs, books, research, developments. One path from here into COVID is a more profound insight into cause and management. Another path is motivation. We are going to need tons of motivation. Where did it come from until now? Will we fare better from now on?

It will start/continue with people saying there is no time for this. [see: "No Time to Waste on Subconceptual Processing"]

But really, it starts with an insight into complexity.

Complexity

Complex is not *complicated*. An engineer can manage something complicated, like a lunar rocket, using numbers and rules and algorithms. Complexity is different from this in its huge amount of degrees of freedom. One can support complexity, but one cannot manage it in the same way as complicatedness. [see: "Complex is not Complicated"]

You cannot make a plant grow by pulling at its leaves.

An organism is complex. A mechanism can be quite complicated without any complexity.

It works until it doesn't anymore

Treating an organism (such as any human being or a crowd) as a mechanism may work initially. 'Motivating' people to stay home, for instance, in corona times. Put some pressure on it (anxiety, guilt, shame), and the first mechanical goal may be reached. People do stay home a bit more to avoid infection. Nice!

The hidden sides are less nice. Anxiety — especially in combination with loneliness, aggression, and many other causes of stress — is a pathogen: it makes people sick through immune dysregulation and many other pathways. Also, anxiety is a negative motivator: it leads to resistance, one way or another. You can see that as a backlash. I like the metaphor of a ball that is pushed underwater. When the pushing abruptly stops, a big splash follows. Reality is more complicated than the metaphor: next time, the ball may resist even more.

Unfortunately, the beginner's success in motivating this way may heighten his conviction that this is the way to go. Unfortunately, we see this happen regularly in corona times. If the ball resists, the pushing needs to get harder. Meanwhile, the splashing around makes the pusher think he's getting more important. After a while, the ball itself becomes the enemy or at least a big part of the problem. The pusher becomes indispensable. Here arises a policy of rules and repression. Unfortunately, we also see this happen in corona times. People are being pushed in different directions. Where has motivation gone?

Jesus!

I'm not your regular Bible-Santa-Christian guy. However, New Testament poetry is adorable — no condescension in this. In my view, that's enough to please any God, whether really real or poetically real. In the end, there is no deeply relevant difference.

The evening before His arrest, Jesus washed the feet of his disciples. Is this an act of servant leadership or not? A few days later, they deserted Him out of fear/anxiety. A few weeks after that, at Pentecost, the disciples received inspiration from above, which made them brave and ready to preach 'in tongues,' this is: using the language of inspiration. Well, it wasn't a flame that did the trick, but the washing of feet.

If you want to be inspiring/motivating as a leader, you have to wash feet. Soap may be nice. It's enough if you do that once and never forget. If you don't forget, others don't forget since they see it alive inside you. You have successfully incorporated it. You are a motivating leader.

This doesn't happen so much. If it happens, it's beautiful!

Motivation – demotivation – manipulation

Human energy = deep motivation. Someone who doesn't have much energy to accomplish something, is just little in-depth motivated. One is not the cause of the other. It's the same thing.

So, we can talk about 'energy' without misunderstanding. People do need it. If you take it away, people will not do what you want them to do. That's called *demotivation*. It's easier than motivation. Anxiety, for instance, is an energy-sucker. It demotivates, especially over time. When even the anxiety-energy gets depleted, people become complacent, as if they don't care anymore for what is ethically right. In reality, they do still care, but the batteries are empty. In corona times, one can see this as seemingly not caring anymore about many unnecessary deaths. Economy first! Own people first! But for what purpose? What is the economy for if not for an ethical goal? [see: "The Final COVID Question: Ethics or Economics?"] What is ethics in the first place if you take out the caring? Nothing.

Demotivated people have lost (contact with) their positive energy. This makes them prone to any manipulation that feeds on their energy from a negative angle. Mind: the energy is still present but in a different guise. The energy itself is not negative, but it is prone to be used this way. If some politician finds the route, there's trouble ahead. Need I be explicit?

One can blame the manipulator, or one can blame the lack of motivation.

Ready for motivating crowds?

One more thing, repeatedly: you cannot motivate. You can only let people be motivated from inside. There is no alternative.

A crowd is a tremendous opportunity for motivation. You can let much of the work be done by crowd activity. Again: People do not motivate other people, but they see others being motivated. That's an effective communication towards inside, an example of empathy through mirroring. So, try to make people see others being motivated. No manipulation, please; you don't have to lie about sizes of crowds. Just don't be coy about favorable reality. As a leader, be proud of what you have accomplished and let people know. They will additionally be motivated by your being proud. Indeed, they'll do their best to make you even prouder. Isn't it gorgeous?

Never forget that, as a leader, your function is also a symbolic one. I hope that, in the future, no leader will ever be able to forget this. It is the main thing a leader 'does.' And at first sight, it's almost nothing. It's Openness. [see: "No Future without Open Leadership"]

See also chapter on 'Leadership in Corona Times.'

From this Openness – and only from here – you can do many things: give people confidence, relieve stress and anxiety while *heightening* motivation through this, let them really care for each other, let them be really grateful, let them be proud to wear a mask, let them think about how each can personally do something positive. Oh, so many things.

Is it a job? Yes, it's a job!

It may seem simple only for one who doesn't know what it's about. It's not simple at all. But it's not necessarily complicated. It's complex.

And that makes it quite some job!

Every piece of communication needs to be motivating. I repeat: Every piece of communication needs to be motivating. You repeat it now, please. You see? It never ends.

Also, it never begins. It's not something clear-cut that you 'do' on top of other things. It should live inside the motivator. He embodies it. He symbolizes it. He grows it inside. Only then can it grow in others.

Is it a job? No, it's much more than a job!

Who's job?

Leadership is everybody's job. Motivation is everybody's job. There is not one person responsible. Everybody's responsible. So, you are clearly responsible. A leader is also responsible because he symbolizes all people to all people. At the symbolic level, if well performed, the leader is the crowd. That is his charisma.

This said, clear job descriptions are mandatory. A scientist is a scientist; a politician is a politician, a representative is a representative. Even a maverick at times should be that: a maverick at times. It's optimal to have them regularly together; it's a sure road to chaos to have them communicate publicly in intermingled ways.

I repeat: Every piece of communication needs to be motivating, especially towards crowds.

By the way: Chaos is not complex. Chaos is just chaos.

Corona motivation

In my view, this should be fully grounded in Compassion. [see: "COVID Compassion"] Compassion is not the same as pity, of course. This said, there's much to be sad about. Many people suffer; many are in burnout or post-traumatic stress. Many are mourning others. Every unnecessary death should not be!

One minute of silence.

Compassion is also an excellent motivator because people can feel it inside. So, how do you get it inside? Certainly not by bickering, nor by showing superficial emotions. Nor by showing your anxiety, nor by showing your incapability to be anxious about the fate of others. Do allow yourself to be anxious if you are, then try to deal with it without getting into active denial. Enacting denial as a window to your hidden anxiety may be one of the strongest demotivators. Don't do it.

You get Compassion by showing Compassion as well as by seeing it in others.

Their finest hour?

At the time of writing, the worldwide situation is awful, and it will get worse.

Living through this together may, after all is said and experienced, be something that people will look back upon as something with excellent aspects. It may be 'their finest hour.' Ring a bell?

Let's make this era something to be proud of, finding proper motivation to carry on. This includes youth, or should I say: those who will think back of this, fifty years from now.

Will they still be grateful then for the support they get (and give) in these most trying times?

Will they have memories to cherish?

29. Our Mind Is Our Way Out (or Into) COVID

October 2, 2020

	Today	Total
Cases worldwide	314.470	34.500.786
Deaths worldwide	5.583	1.027.136

COVID is a mind-body problem. Most experts in the picture are not mind-body experts.
▶ ▶ ▶ We use our mind appropriately and get out of the worst troubles, or we don't and we don't. ◀ ◀ ◀

Too little, too late

This text is another try as a wake-up call, being urgent and partially too late by now. Too late sadly for many people as well as to prevent the wave that is about to rack several economies, including some of the countries who wanted to put lives and ethics first. I see this, for instance, in the case of Argentina. It's heartbreaking.

Who is going to communicate – too late – that it is to some extent, perhaps even largely preventable by properly using our mind?

The economy: simple

Although the economy cannot tolerate another lockdown, it will get beaten worse in the coming twelve months than in the previous. We will go into another lockdown precisely because we desperately want to avoid lockdown "for the economy cannot take it." So, we will wait too long.

Again.

This is because the next year will be amazingly (unsuspectedly, even today) horrendous. Some 'turbo phenomenon' will come as if from nowhere.

Predictably amazingly.

Why?

Mind: complex

Arguably, around half of this mayhem is due to conceptual, virus-related factors.

The other half is due to mind-related factors. To be precise, these are subconceptual. One can approximate this with the term nonconscious. For instance, one cannot consciously decide to be immune to panic. One cannot consciously choose to have a placebo effect. One cannot consciously decide to be motivated to wear a face mask, nor to anything else. Our conscious motivation is not a cause, but a side effect, as is so little known in public and so much in proper science.

One cannot consciously decide to influence one's immune system, good or bad. Yet nonconsciously, there is a huge and scientifically validated influence, as is again (much too) little known in public. This public includes many physicians.

Mind→body influences are much more complex as well as – accordingly – much more significant than is generally thought, especially in medicine at the level of practitioners.

Meanwhile, the highest-level science shows many such mind-body influences, as I expanded upon in MINDING COVID and other books and articles. Now I put the starkly naked conclusion as the title of this blog/chapter.

Seasonality is almost certain.

Never say 100%. Well, 98%.

Surprisingly perhaps, the seasonality of infectious disease is still little understood. We know a few interfering factors. The mind also plays an important role. It is undoubtedly not only virus-related + a matter of people staying indoors.

With seasonality, we are already feeling autumn in Europe. I see in this the temptative debut of the second wave. Winter will be bad.

Comes the COVID whirlpool.

Whirlpool

Since one doesn't see nonconscious mind, it is not there...? Hmm, although this thinking is prevalent worldwide, it still is the thinking of a preschooler.

Driven also by nonconscious mental elements, the COVID whirlpool is ready to strike again, the big way. Don't just believe me but, at least, think like an adult. We need to be fearful without getting anxious. Denial makes people prone to tumble into the whirlpool at the moment of unavoidable truth. It is a lousy defense against panic.

With the possibility of repeat infections by SARS-CoV-2 being a certainty by now, and expected to become the rule rather than the exception, reaching herd immunity gets more complicated (https://www.scientificamerican.com/article/what-covid-19-reinfection-means-for-vaccines). We need every possible support, conceptually and subconceptually. The whirlpool is a bad thing, but insight in it can provide additional means to escape it.

Virologists, etc.

In my country (Belgium) and worldwide, virologists have hardly an inkling about nonconscious processing. They have no training in this. They didn't become virologists because they were aficionados of the psyche from the start. Quite the contrary, some are the most mind-body aversive people, thus inhibiting rather than enhancing this side of the solution. These experts are not experts in mind-body.

So, they are understandably suspicious of mind-body within a culture that is as a whole weary of mind-body. It is indeed difficult to see one's thinking as influential on the body within a double emergence [body → mind → consciousness]. Yet it is our reality as human beings, not as bodies devoid of mind, and mind – never mind. Bizarre?

From a mere consciousness-viewpoint, indeed, it is bizarre. If you look at it from a reality-viewpoint, the picture changes dramatically.

Patients do not exist for the sake of medicine.

But meanwhile, these experts guide politics, which is OK. In mind-body matters, they do so abysmally, which is not OK. Of course, they are not guilty. Mud-throwing is out of the question. Objectivity is of utmost importance in science. This is one more reason why science should not act politically. It should support and guide politics. In this, it should also be broad, not narrowly self-serving.

People do not exist for the sake of science.

Also, science, in its objectivity, is a worldwide undertaking. That takes time, and there is not enough time in COVID-times. Yet the endeavor should remain the same.

"People may not be ready for this,"

as my first publisher warned me twenty years ago. They still may not. Yet, sorry, I think we are in an emergency now. It is less important whether people are ready than it is mandatory to act upon this emergency correctly, even if it hurts some general preconception.

The war metaphor is also deficient in this respect. Did you ever see a war in which those who say "There is no enemy" or worse, "We are our own enemy" are regarded with benevolence? I have been encountering this since March.

We need a Copernican revolution, not putting the earth out of center in the universe, but our ego out of center in our inner universe. I suspect that both are quite related.

Motivation

Mind is also crucial for motivation. As already mentioned, to-be-motivated is not merely a conscious choice. It is a nonconscious happening/action.

We will need motivation to do the right thing concerning COVID, as long as the West is democratic. Either we use our mind, or – very arguably – we might better get authoritarian. Democracy is something to be earned continuously.

We think we have the virus better under control now than in the spring.

Indeed, but it is ourselves that we need to get 'under control' most of all. As with the first wave, we will be the primary source of whirlpool energy. That is not the domain of any mind-less medic. People are never mind-less. However, from historical causes, people have been and are being treated this way.

COVID is a mind-body problem. We need mind-body experts, but we don't have them in place.

Go 200 years in the past: procedures such as blood-letting would be the answer to COVID. It would be the overall accepted thing to do, and blatantly wrong. Indeed, any other therapy from then would be blatantly wrong. By then, the authoritative galenic medicine had been wrong for 1600 years. Oh yes. Oh yes. It is very well possible to flow along in the wrong direction *en masse*. Not surprisingly, since such a flow is particularly strong. [see: "Streaming Underneath"]

Not everything was bleak. A sensible measure from centuries ago and what we still do is quarantine.

"But now we have science!" Indeed, but we don't have any strong mind-body science. In this domain, relatively little relevant progress has been made.

When will we know?

This is preventable, as will be shown some years from now, through real-world evidence. What do we have to wait for? An appropriate use of A.I. tools.

In that same future, *stress* within a population (not only the sum of individuals) will be seen as a crucial issue. It has a considerable impact on health and wellbeing. We need a much better view of what *stress* is in the first place: what concept is relevant, how can it be delineated, what do we care to call *stress*?

Meanwhile, I am troubled by many researchers who don't come out of their comfort zone. This is about more than reluctance. It is an active evasion that I would like to better understand.

What I want?

Most of all, I want to have the means to enable further development, translations, and divulgence of the free app. Of course, I would also like to get the message out. To get rich of all this – COVID and much more – is not wanted unless it's the only way to succeed.

You and I and all know what is at stake. It deeply hurts that developing countries will eventually be the main victims, while the rich are more responsible and need to use our brains – pun totally intended.

This text is not a complaint against anyone.

But I do hope something can be achieved.

30. COVID: <u>Why</u> Hiding the Mind?

October 9, 2020

	Today	Total
Cases worldwide	348.774	36.738.833
Deaths worldwide	6.424	1.066.412

Since March, I have tried to focus medical colleagues and other people on the mind in COVID progression, as yet to little avail. This is utterly weird.

Weirdness

Imagine being as convinced as I am that optimally lending attention to mind→COVID is probably the best we can do, given that a strict population-wide quarantine is not possible in the West. Imagine, meanwhile, having written a book about it, based on other books of mine and a doctorate. Then, the fact that, worldwide, no attention goes to mind→COVID may usher you into a sense of utter weirdness.

Welcome.

Mind?

'Mind' is the totality of mental processing in a human being, consciously and nonconsciously. Scientifically, there is no doubt that mental processing is mostly of the second kind. Yet society worldwide – perhaps particularly in the West – is organized in the sense of not taking this into account.

Of course, one cannot consciously decide to have a mental influence on disease progression, such as COVID. In AURELIS-talk: There is no 'Inner Strength' in consciousness. This may be a significant reason why there is no mind→COVID in the general picture. Indeed:

Without nonconscious processing, it would be a preposterous idea.

But it is not. Contrary to this, it makes the COVID reality that we are living through preposterous in many ways.

The broader picture is that there is supposedly little mind in anything health-related. [see: "The Problem with Corona is the Problem with Medicine"] This makes the COVID case less weird, but only within a much broader field of weirdness.

Trying to ignore the nonconscious within an ever more complex society with ever more complex technology leads to ever weirder situations. This is much more dangerous than even the virus. It pervades healthcare, education, and more. Even politics: conservatives versus progressives. They will never understand each other without delving into the importance of nonconscious processing.

Then why hiding the mind?

This is about more than simply ignoring the mind. It is something more active, which I still don't get very well. It is an anxiety that may show itself quite aggressively sometimes.

In any case, if it would only be an intellectual issue, it would have been resolved already, in three steps:

- Take the above.
- Say: "Hey, guys, the reality is such, not so."
- Problem resolved.

But it isn't.

Some usual suspects

Innate in a human being – indeed, any complex organism – is the propensity to look for the concrete. Abstract thinking is more complicated and less pragmatic if your job is to survive here and now. Conscious processing is more concrete; nonconscious processing, by nature, is less visible. It requires abstract thinking to think about the nonconscious, although it is spontaneously active every day, all day long.

In a way, it is so spontaneously active that it becomes transparent, like glasses that you wear and you forget most of the time that you are wearing them. Looking right through them, it is difficult to see them. [see: "The Basic Cognitive Illusion"]

People generally tend to go with the flow, in a conservative way, especially in times of stress. The present is, of course, a time of stress for many people.

For many, there is status and money involved. Never to be underestimated.

A very broad perspective

This may be the main reason for hiding/ignoring the mind, related to the fundamental nature of mind itself and how it has evolved regarding attention (awareness).

After a very long time in the history of evolution, we are heading towards a 'third wave' of attention in which mere-ego is no longer at center play. Instead, we can cultivate open awareness in which one acts as a total person. Viewed from 'second wave' (with much disregard of nonconscious processing), this provokes an extraordinary amount of anxiety. Without proper support at a grand scale, this may become much more pronounced than it already is. [see: "Three Waves of Attention"]

Humanity may not even survive the transition.

Fortunately, with proper support, the picture changes dramatically. For instance, in COVID, my personal (intuitively, not scientifically based) assessment is that we can still attain a vast diminishment of the disaster that lies ahead, even with only some of the support that I am talking about.

But we are where we are.

This anxiety becomes a prime source of energy within the COVID whirlpool that racks immune systems and economies. The same anxiety also inhibits many people from adequately dealing with the transition. This is a vicious circle by itself. The more intensely people resist it, the more it creates anxiety and stress, so they resist even more.

Many resist even the sight of it in COVID and more. They actively hide when there's a slight chance of making full contact with inner (nonconscious) self.

Very sorry, but this looks like a rabbit seeking refuge from a fox inside a paper bag when the fox is already inside the bag.

31. COVID Management at Society Level

October 18, 2020

	Today	Total
Cases worldwide	372.553	39.939.292
Deaths worldwide	5.567	1.114.196

I bring together elements discussed in previous blogs/chapters to show that reckoning with the deeper mind and the COVID-whirlpool may lead to specific society-wide (polity) measures that – on top of common-sense hygienic measures – may lessen the pending calamity.

Complexity

Some insight in complexity is advisable. [see: "Complex is not Complicated"]

In the COVID-whirlpool [see: "COVID-Whirlpool"], physical and mental elements reinforce each other and thus can – as a whole – have a much more significant influence than the sum of the elements. Looking at separate components, one cannot grasp the total happening, leading to surprises time and again. This general phenomenon is a characteristic of any complex system. In COVID, it is crucial at the individual and societal level.

On top of this, in the COVID case, many mental elements are subconceptual. This leads to being hardly visible — amazingly (yes, even now, still, to me) worldwide. I see in the cause of this a confluence of intrapsychic and social factors. Of course, they intermingle, additionally fuel the COVID-whirlpool.

Two causal results of this additional social fuel

Individual and societal:

- For the individual, it is even harder to keep out of the danger zone. In several personal experiences, I see people just let themselves flow towards it. They don't resist. Drifting on a social stream, it's stronger than themselves: <Do as thy neighbor.> Probably – and I fear very much for this – increasingly, many people will get into the situation in which they give it up *and are even glad to give it up*. Thus, many people prefer to live in denial of inconvenient truths: "I'll see when I get sick. Before that, I don't want to make my life miserable. I want to live a pretty normal life." In this way, one may think to be in comfortable control, while disaster is nearby, occurring more rapidly and effectively than expected. Leadership is supposed to bring this comfortable control.

- Yet in due time, at the society level, measures fall over measures, going from one ineffective situation to the next, from insupportable lockdown to throwing all open, to communicating the impossibility of a subsequent lockdown until it is the only way to proceed. Meanwhile, in a society with 'free' vocalization, a huge cacophony self-perpetuates critiques about every measure from the moment things go wrong.

What to do?

Let's look at some examples and learn some lessons. Main lesson: It is possible, at the society level, to exert an immense influence upon our COVID future.

Looking at Uruguay

Inhabitants: 3.5 million

Deaths per million up to now: 15.

New cases today: 30.

South-America as a continent is faring poorly on COVID. This makes Uruguay (and Paraguay) an interesting case, an island of COVID health despite its having the highest percentage of aged 65+ of the continent. They had no forced lockdown. This resembles Japan, for instance, where the number of COVID-related deaths is even lower. It is possible, also in a democracy!

The Uruguayan government took early and severe measures: quarantine, closing schools, and big shopping malls, demanding an early use of face masks. They also used innovative technologies: own diagnostic tests and early contact tracing, excellent information of the public through mobile apps, chatbots, and social media.

They used good sensibilization campaigns, brought from an advising committee of scientists in coordination with the private sector. All went with relatively high transparency. A mobile app, 'Coronavirus UY,' enables the following of cases. A coronavirus fund transparently allocates the money spent. In general, the government is open in what, why, how things are done. There is even a temporary diminishment of the pay of the president, ministers, and best-paid administrators. This all leads to a high level of social cohesion. Trust in the government made people motivated to follow the guidelines

Looking at Vietnam

Inhabitants: 97,6 million

Deaths per million up to now: 0,4.

New cases today: 6.

According to observers, Vietnam has put in place superb public-health communication. From very early on (second week of January), an alert of pending danger went to the public. In February, the government was advocating for social distancing and hand-washing. In April, a fine for social media posts of false information was installed.

These logical steps inspired, from early on, every citizen to do their part: wearing masks, weeks of quarantine, etc.

Vietnam, a relatively poor country, totals less COVID deaths until now than there are every 90 minutes in the US.

Looking at Belgium

Reluctantly, since we are one of the worst performing countries regarding COVID.

Inhabitants: 11,6 million

Deaths per million up to now: 897

New cases today: 10.964

This is thought-provoking, at least. The cacophony is massive. Lots of anxiety and worn-out people, including health professionals. Guidelines to the public are chaotically inconsistent and each time overshadowed by critique. Everybody knows everything and nothing, inundating media. I don't even know – nor do I care – how many governmental health departments we have in this small country with room for one.

There is much empathy, but in its short-sightedness, it adds to the problem. Here is way too much short-sighted empathy and too little Compassion. That is a recipe for troubles in any country of the free world.

Too late in Europe and the US?

A therapeutic roundup: progress has been made mainly in organ support. Corticoids are obvious. Killer-medications have not been developed. A vaccine may bring relief, little and late. This makes it *impossible* for some countries to break through the bad times and proceed without a renewed lockdown. As before, in a direct way, the West will suffer much more than the East.

For instance, in the US, key coronavirus forecasts predict over 410,000 total deaths by Jan. 1. In case of little compliance with simple measures, this can reach as high as 620,000. [https://www.cnbc.com/2020/09/04/key-coronavirus-forecast-predicts-over-410000-total-us-deaths-by-jan-1.html#close] In fact, there is quite some skepticism about projections extending this far into the future because there are many unknown factors. Reassuring? One such factor is how the virus's spread may be affected by the changing seasons. The most important factor that can change the outcome of an outbreak is how humans respond. People's behavior changes over time and is essentially unpredictable.

Projections of deaths worldwide also vary widely, according to compliance to simple measures. [https://covid19.healthdata.org/global?view=total-deaths&tab=trend]: February 21, 2021:

Mandates easing	3.496.912
Current projection	2.418.545
Universal masks	1.800.406

We will get out of it in the spring, most probably, somehow,

and then – don't be surprised – it will happen again as long as the invisible (our deep mind) is not clearly in focus. We're talking about 2021, 2022, and so on.

What about the economy? What about the human COVID-suffering? What about indirect morbidity and mortality, deaths by famine worldwide? The social and political unrest, and everything involved in that?

The subconceptual is necessary in management at the society level

Between fearmongering and active denial, there is a space of common sense.

Since the virus is with us, the more infected people stay out of the COVID-whirlpool, the better the community will fare in the end, and with a fairly decent economy. Respecting the mind – conceptually and subconceptually – will help us stay out of the whirlpool and attain herd immunity with or without vaccination.

Several chapters are about what this means individually (about the app and so on). Let's focus now on society and social polity. A country that doesn't get the subconceptual right is at risk of going down until a miracle vaccine or medication appears.

Therefore, at every level, COVID should be managed with conceptual as well as subconceptual insight. The latter is, among other things, about people's trust in leadership and each other. If people are thus motivated, much less hard rules and lockdowns are needed.

A basic rule can be as follows:

People – individuals – need to know, "I can handle this."

'To know' is not only objective but also about being deeply convinced. I will repeatedly use the term 'deep.' [see also: "Deep Motivation"]

'This' is what is meaningful, or, indeed, deeply meaningful.

All else depends on this essential knowing. It can be realized through one's strength or with proper support from the trusted leadership. One feels confident and also sees others being confident. Thus, each individual is confident that others will do what is needed to get over the challenge. Either they are forced or deeply motivated. In any case, people need to trust each other in doing the right thing.

So, pointing out that a particular subgroup doesn't follow the rules and that everybody needs to follow these rules to prevent disaster is to be avoided. For example, a well-meaning communication is the following:

> "People need to do five simple things. If they do these things, then everything is OK, and we will be fine."

This is a clear and motivating message that puts people at ease and in control.

Is it?

In a 'free country,' it puts guilt on people. Let me rephrase:

"If you don't do these simple things that any child can do, it will not 'be fine.' The disaster that we foresee will be your fault or the fault of those who don't comply, and you can do nothing about it. We are all trapped like rats in a cage. Surely, 'they' are to blame."

Telling people they should be motivated is not a right way.

Telling someone to be motivated is not motivating. How could it be? To become motivated is not a conscious act. To think it is, is part of our basic cognitive illusion, ubiquitously wrongfully present. [see: "The Basic Cognitive Illusion"]

Telling people that it's easy to prevent further COVID mishap, "just following some basic rules," doesn't instill confidence, especially if people see others not following the rules already for a long time. Contrary to this, solidarity should be enhanced in every possible way, not by saying that it should be done, but by pointing to the why, time and again. The why, well-articulated, invites people to grow to the occasion, time and again. People may need to be invited many times.

People also need to know they are on the same side as their leadership. Most important is not that everybody agrees with the measurements – which would be impossible anyway – but that all share the same end-values. It is about the articulated 'why.' You see: People need to know they can handle this. Therefore, of course, it needs to be the right this, the one they recognize to be relevant to them.

For this purpose, regular (daily) communications are a must. This should be seen as part of COVID management itself. People need to see their leader's efforts. It relieves stress and impacts COVID straight on. COVID is treated by doctors *and* by leaders.

Isn't it beautiful, after all?

The war metaphor

may be efficient to unite people, but it has substantial negative sides, especially since 'the enemy' is invisible in COVID. Inside an individual's brain/mind, the pattern of associations around 'enemy' may look for a visible alternative. In the end, everybody can be infectious, so everybody can be 'the enemy.'

The war metaphor can be active because people may have much pent-up energy. This may get a better outlet in 'fighting' without the need for war or aggression. People's fighting *for* each other unites them in better ways. Without this outlet, it may be challenging to detract the metaphorical thinking about war. It may even be quite stressful. It may give the impression of making yourself and others vulnerable.

This includes the 'warriors,' the healthcare workers, especially those who are in a warrior mindset by nature. Many are; many are not. Those who are can act fiercely against any hint of an alternative take.

Healthcare workers need deep respect.

They don't need white cloths on window sills.

How do they get deep respect? How does anyone get deep respect? White cloth may have this intention. It may also show deep respect, but not necessarily.

If leadership regularly mentions healthcare workers, for instance, when admonishing people to social distancing, that's already one step further. It brings people together with healthcare workers and each other in deep meaningfulness. Little ads on television can significantly help.

> "With THIS, you prevent THIS."

> "On top of their regular job, they care for you. Please care for them."

If healthcare workers feel deep respect also without the cloths, then the cloths start to really become meaningful.

Valuing life is always motivating in any communication.

Such as:

> "We value the life of old people. We also value their quality of life. There are important differences in how old individuals value their life versus its quality. So we want to give them a choice to the degree of what is possible."

This is a deep communication. If coming from the heart, it is 'deep to deep.' There's something energetic in this. It is charismatic. It is graceful. It is a present of inner beauty.

It is the ultimate <u>this</u> to be handled. It is ultimately meaningful.

What is 'life' to you?

32. COVID: Still Flying on One Wing

October 30, 2020

	Today	Total
Cases worldwide	545.945	45.313.410
Deaths worldwide	7.172	1.185.738

Mad man

We're at the end of October, in full autumn by now. As I wrote months ago, we're in full autumn-COVID, which comes before winter-COVID in Europe and the US.

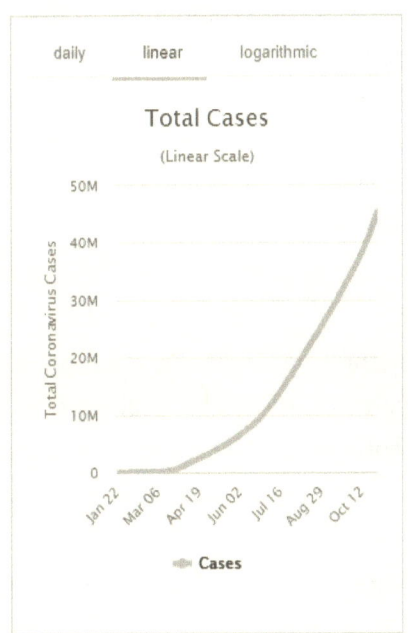

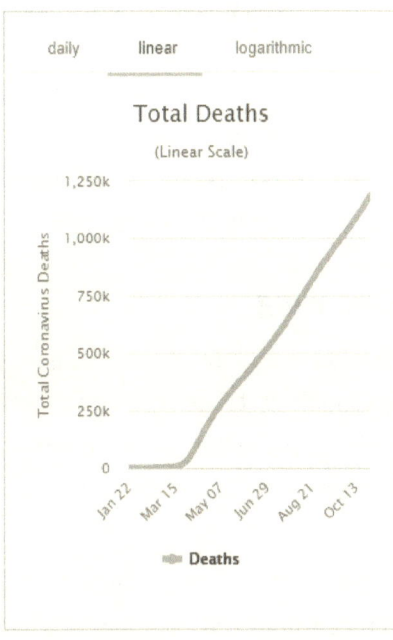

I was going to be (somewhat) angry, and that's what I am, looking at the curves of worldwide cases and deaths from https://www.worldometers.info/coronavirus/. Total cases go up with testing capacity as well as with the number of infections. The testing capacity has increased very much since springtime. Thus, by itself, 'total cases' is a controversial metric, as are others, but they all point in one direction.

Total deaths

Deaths can hardly be faked. Are they all COVID-caused? That's difficult to say. There is no uni-causality in many deaths, generally. Does someone with a precondition + COVID die from COVID or his precondition? Without the precondition, he would not have died. So?

An indicator can be found in excess deaths within a period in 2020 as compared to the same period in 2019. Quoting CDC: "Overall, an estimated 299,028 excess deaths occurred from late January through October 3, 2020, with 198,081 (66%) excess deaths attributed to COVID-19." [https://www.cdc.gov/mmwr/volumes/69/wr/mm6942e2.htm]

Compare this with what you may. To me, every preventable death is, well, preventable; therefore, relevant. Moreover, what is not incorporated in the graphic is the ongoing and pending amount of deaths through indirect causes: famine, violence, lack of medical support in developing countries, among other things a diminishing degree of vaccinations for other diseases. Most COVID-related deaths will be indirect this way.

One wing

As you know by now, I mean with this that only the conceptually graspable is taken into account. Meanwhile, of course, reality doesn't care about what is or is not conceptually graspable. It is fully our responsibility to see through this. Flying on two wings can make it a very different story.

It is an immense responsibility. On the other hand, it is also an immensely difficult undertaking, mainly because it is counter-cultural and leads to essential changes in mind-related domains. Interestingly, every human field is mind-related. This shows the need to reconsider many givens and preconceptions, some of which are millennia-old. That looks daunting, and it is.

It's daunting and unrealized, also in COVID's fields.

The consequence is our flying on merely the conceptual wing. The other wing is what I call 'subconceptual.' This is the subject of my Ph.D. and a lot of further research and development. The relevance is diverse: a direct mind-body influence on COVID progression (as there is on other viral diseases), a more specifically COVID-related 'staying out of the whirlpool' [see: "COVID-Whirlpool"] other psychological and psycho-somatic consequences, human motivation (to wear a mask, to get vaccinated).

As to motivation, indeed, note that this has also traditionally been regarded from a conceptual viewpoint. But can you in conscious awareness decide to be motivated for anything? Amazingly not. [see: "Non-Conscious Processing is Meaningful"] Motivation is basically non-conscious and subconceptual, which is, of course, why it's also such a conundrum to many leaders, teachers, and physicians. That is difficult to grasp for many, but, again, reality doesn't care for this difficulty.

Deeper self

The 'deeper self' may be an eyebrow-lifting term to some, as it is to me. By lack of a better term, I use it to denote the scientifically evidenced way that our brain works. Through this, one can best comprehend mind-body-unity. It is, shortly put, the mental/neuronal pattern level. [see: "Human Brain: Giant Pattern Recognizer"] Scientific progress in this field is evolving rapidly and is extremely promising in that it gradually shows what is, for instance, the meaning of 'meaning' at the brain level.

Through this, the 'deeper self' is becoming visible from the neuronal side. We also get a better view of the huge implications of non-conscious processing. This has been hinted on for centuries before S. Freud, who wrote about the 'subconscious' in an unfortunately quite conceptual way at the start of the 20th century. We know much more about subconceptual processing at present, in many ways.

We lack robust experimental science about the mental perspective on the same. The psychological research is still flawed, leading to a crisis in the reproducibility of prior high-level scientific experiments. This is not surprising since our scientific instruments are made to investigate the conceptual, not the subconceptual. This is relevant mainly in view of the complexity of the latter. [see: "Complex is not Complicated"]

When will this change?

I guess, in a few years from now. Technology, mainly A.I.-driven, will help. [see: "Dawn of Opening Up"] One way or another, this technology will result in real-world evidence.

Sadly, it will be too late to prevent the present disaster. But this is not the end of the world, nor the human species. Challenges abound, to which this dawn is the beginning. Let's hope it will all proceed well. Compassion will be central to the direction of humanity, and even of intelligence on this planet and more.

Wow. The future is a long time. Meanwhile, in a few years already, on condition that the right choices are made, we will investigate and understand much better the influence of our mind (deeper self) on something like COVID progression.

Dear reader, if you read this in the future, please take a minute to think about 2020 in this vein.

Thanks.

On one wing, the second wing is rather a nuisance.

In the case of COVID, it shows as nocebo in being a primary cause of the COVID-whirlpool, individually and as a society. [see: "Is Social Nocebo Real?"] We know nocebo can be substantial in other domains. The subconceptual is powerful in a positive and negative direction.

It also shows in the whole field of psycho-somatics, in the present-day mind-negating stance called 'MUS.' [see: "Medically Unexplained

Syndromes (MUS)"] Even with the blunt instruments of now, we see a considerable influence of 'distress' on many health issues. We see – already – the relevance of depression, anxiety, loneliness, and chronic aggression on physical symptoms and disease. All of them are relevant in COVID-times.

Mad men

Understandably, many caregivers are cross. They have to work in trying circumstances and even at the peril of their own lives. Many have post-traumatic stress or even burnout, visible especially if one cares to see through the veil. They, too, should know and mind about nocebo. Also, there are many socio-relational problems for caregivers, personally. The continuous idea that this situation could have been largely prevented is, understandably, hard to take.

This will not evolve positively throughout the winter.

Personally,

with insight into my own research, I see even more how it could have been prevented. Sadly, this is still going on in full glory. I don't get my ideas inside the heads of many. There is too much streaming underneath. [see: "Streaming Underneath"]

So I'm finishing up a few things in November, such as a hands-on concrete corpus and groundwork for Lisa [see: "Lisa"]. The COVID situation will be a lot worse in December than it is now, especially through not recognizing the second wing. Many medical colleagues will be on the brink. That's the time for me also to take my responsibility as a physician. Hopefully, I can combine it with fieldwork concerning 'Minding Corona.' After that, we'll see.

33. Can Mind Acutely Prevent COVID?

November 1, 2020

	Today	Total
Cases worldwide	475.201	46.367.473
Deaths worldwide	6.488	1.199.727

Can the mind acutely play a role in the timeframe between getting a sufficient quantity of the virus inside your body and COVID: either showing symptoms or becoming asymptomatically infectious?

Answers depend on how you pose questions.

Without changing reality by simply posing some questions, one can change a line of research. For seven COVID-related months, I have been thinking that the title's question wasn't worth bothering.

Now, I do.

Warning and disclaimer

From March 2020 onwards, I deemed a mind-influence on COVID to be so evident that it's silly not to research it. Bringing scientific elements together, as in *MINDING CORONA*, any clear-thinking researcher would acknowledge. The problem is that, as far as I know, none care or dare to look into this direction.

The title's question is new. I didn't care or dare to pose it myself until now. My failure. Science is not only about experiments. It's also about daring to keep thinking. Still, this is somewhat hypothetical. Please make up your mind on the evidence.

Viral load, viral shedding

One gets sick or infectious when having *many* viruses in the body, not just a few. However, one can get infected by a relatively low amount. The viruses replicate and keep on replicating exponentially. Then they inundate a person who gets sick either by the sheer amount of viruses destroying cells or by an overreaction of the defense system. In principle, one can get very ill or die from both.

Meanwhile, viral load (the amount of viruses in the body) is one factor in viral shedding (the amount of viruses that one spreads around). Thus, viral load is essential in infectiousness even from before symptoms appear. But first:

Minding immunity

The mind quite heavily influences the immune system. Actually, it has become apparent – science, you know – that the immune system and the central nervous system work together in forming the mind. This is:

> You think – up to some degree – with your immune system.

Makes you think, no?

Then the question is:

Can the immune system, influenced by the mind, affect viral load from early on, say, a few days after the arrival of our little guests? Thus, can the mind enhance or prevent illness and reduce infectiousness from early on?

Can the mind act so quickly on immunology? That would be impressive. On the other hand, with still relatively little viral load, a small influence might be enough.

Let us pause for a coffee.

Right. If the mind can be harnessed profoundly within the specified timeframe, then as a procedure combined with rapid mass testing and a few days of quarantine, the COVID problem can melt like snow on a warm and sunny day. Hurray!

Even if the effect is relatively small, it's already substantial — and interestingly far-reaching.

Possibly relevant to COVID?

Most people do not get sick after infestation with corona. In many cases, we don't know why. Even where we have part of an explanation, a large gap exists where the mind can be an important factor. If this explanatory gap would be totally filled with mind, then we should better see the virus as no more than a key to the door.

"We don't know if the mind plays a central role" should not get translated into "We know that the mind does not play a central role." Yet this kind of reasoning is what we see in many other health-related domains.

To be possible, there should be the possibility of a rapid influence of mind on our defense systems. For this, our defense systems themselves need to be able to respond quickly. Of course, they do. The quickest response is innate and nonspecific. There are two lines in this:

1) Enzymes in epithelia (such as the walls of the upper and lower respiratory system), mucus consistency, cough reflex
2) Many precursor immune cells are available from early on in life. These are slightly or not specific but <u>fast</u>. We know much about their existence.

Do you sometimes get a dry mouth from being emotional? That's part of 1). Also, lots of mind-immune influences are known in many ways. It would be surprising if there would not be a substantial influence on 2). One indication is the effect of stress on the efficiency of vaccination.

About complexity: The immune system is immensely complex, and so is the mind. [see= "Complex is not Complicated"] In complexity, relevant reactions can be spontaneous and quick. There is no need for a lot of mathematics in the brain. Elements of a complex system work in parallel to give almost immediate results. Think of the letter 'A.' All right. How long did it take you? Now think, "Hmm, this may be interesting, after all." See? The latter assertion is quite complex. Did it take much time and effort? No.

Another example: A straight guy sees an attractive woman → His pupils may dilate within 300 milliseconds. This is before a conscious reaction is even possible. Note that this is emotionally meaning-driven and quite a complex feat by that guy's brain. Also noteworthy is the absent role of consciousness. The non-conscious mind is very complex and meaning-driven. That is the point I want to make.

As an example of direct immune influence, look at allergies. Immune reactions in the domain of allergy are immediate. Being allergic to a flower, the smell of the flower can quickly lead to the start of immune responses, even an asthma attack.

> Indeed, even if it is a plastic flower, as studies show. This is mental: the idea that a specific flower-allergen is present. This would seem weird, where it not that we already know that the mind and immune system work closely together. The brain-immune-system recognizes the pattern 'flower.' Flower-allergens (physical) are part of this pattern. Apparently, the mental side is also enough to kindle the same pattern into action. [see: "So plastic flowers are real after all... are they?"]

It is possible and even probable that the mind acutely influences our defenses against the virus. Indeed, why would nature NOT do this? It is perfectly capable, and this makes sense.

What about nocebo?

Nocebo is a negative effect stemming from the idea that a negative effect will be. It is a reverse placebo. So, may we be imbuing people with nocebo in the field of COVID?

We put people in quarantine, an acute stress situation, with the message that "bad things may come." Some people are more susceptible than others, especially after a history of chronic stress (such as months of anxiety). The result: A stress-shock on an already chronically stressed organism may give the virus its chance to replicate. That is nocebo.

This does not mean that we can and must prevent all nocebo. We have to put it in the balance. And maybe we can do something to diminish this nocebo. Just wait for a few paragraphs.

Nocebo into whirlpool at this stage?

Another crucially important question about the nocebo-effect: Can it be present within the COVID-whirlpool in an asymptomatic patient? Remember that this whirlpool is a self-enhancing pattern of mutually reinforcing elements. [see: "COVID-Whirlpool - In Which Virus AND Mind Play Substantial Roles"] Can this play a role without symptoms?

I guess the question will be answered entirely in the future. For now, note that an asymptomatic patient does not *consciously* show symptoms. Of course, body-mind does not only react to what is conscious. Much research indicates that what happens at the conscious level is only the tip of the iceberg. Physiological things of which there is non-conscious awareness in the brain are happening in the body before the patient reports symptoms. Note also that placebo/nocebo is a non-consciously caused phenomenon. [see: "Power of Placebo < Autosuggestion"] With all effort in the world, one cannot 'merely consciously will' a placebo-effect into existence. One also cannot 'merely consciously will' to oneself an allergic reaction.

Thus, in principle, non-conscious elements can be part of the whirlpool also in asymptomatic patients. Moreover, there is a gradual transition from symptoms being non-consciously present towards more conscious awareness. Can the brain associate what is happening in the body at this early stage and 'danger ahead'? Well, can the brain-immune-system do so? Yes, this is how new body-alien elements are detected in a whole range of immunology. It is business as usual.

All elements are present for a whirlpool starting at the asymptomatic stage. It must be a little whirlpool, but little is needed at this stage to make a huge difference in the outcome.

Moreover, in my view, the whole COVID-whirlpool is driven by non-conscious elements, even if several are also consciously present. This approaches the philosophical question of consciousness as an epiphenomenon.

Why is all this not already scientifically investigated, apparent, known?

It is implicit, covert, subconceptual, complex. This is not being taught in medical school. I say 'not,' indeed, meaning *absolutely nothing*.

Why is the mind not present in the whole COVID story? [see: "COVID: Why Hiding the Mind?"] The modern medical view on the human being – in body and mind – is a mechanical one. That way, it's hardly possible to see the acute influence of the mind. The mind has no impact as a *mechanical* thing. It has an impact as a *complex* thing. There is an immense difference between the two.

Ask any random virologist about 'deeply meaningful mental (subconceptual) processing' and behold the blank stare. More broadly, merely-conceptual medical specialists are simply the wrong specialists in this subdomain. If only these guided us, we would get where, unfortunately, we are. The issue is not a viral one. It is a virus-mind-body one.

Without whining about the past, we should take action towards the future.

AURELIS mental exercises to prevent COVID

I have made ten relevant, meditative exercises and put them on the app as a new domain. Please, read the warning and disclaimer above again. Scientific experimental research is possible. If you want to help the AURELIS project and yourself, enabling things such as this research, please subscribe.

These mental exercises are in the genre of what is already available on the free app. [see: "Free App to Relieve COVID"] Who would want to do these exercises? Anybody who wants to reduce (not necessarily obliterate) his risk of getting ill, some risk of dying, and being infectious to others. Many people might say 'no' to this. Many others might say 'yes.'

Note that these exercises are not in any way *positive thinking*. Here, the 'locus of control' lies in conscious processing while the non-conscious is regarded as some mechanism to be used by the one in control, being the 'ego.' [see: "The Story of Ego"] AURELIS reaches far beyond. It gets going where positive thinking ends. In respect for the total person (conscious, non-conscious), logically, it is more effective to work with the totality. Otherwise, you risk an inner battle of opposing motivations. Given human complexity, I don't think that one can manipulate oneself into beating the virus. Mr. Tough-guy may even have a contrary effect.

It's better to strive for alignment. AURELIS mental exercises are available to support you, not to do it for you. You can see these new exercises as a diminishment of nocebo and a garnering of your non-conscious mental processing in a healthy way at a time when you need it.

34. Millions of Unneeded COVID Deaths in 2021?

What do you think?
December 12, 2020

	Daily	Total
Cases worldwide	704.570	71.454.215
Deaths worldwide	12.413	1.600.483

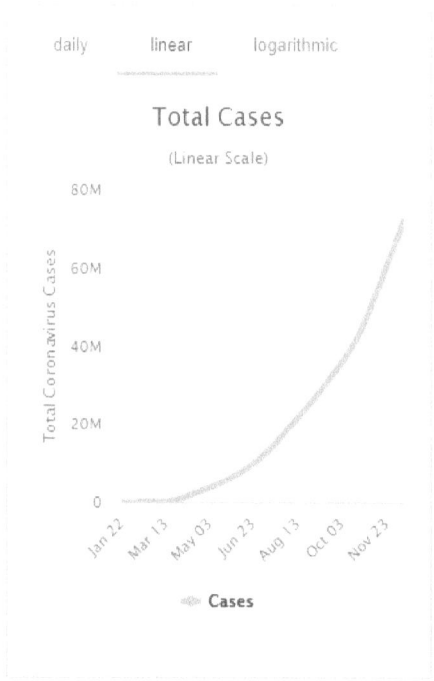

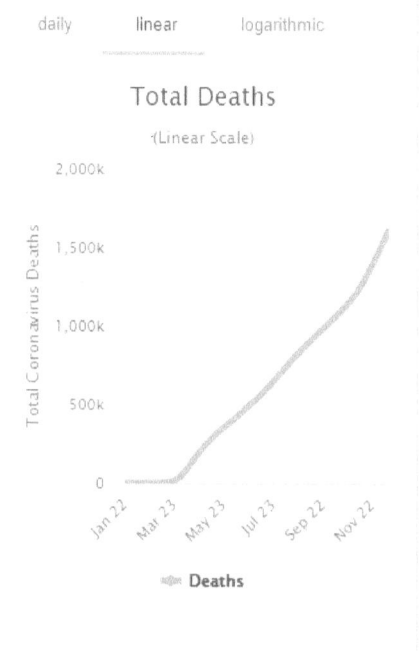

(https://www.worldometers.info)

Nobody dies with no reason.

There is always a reason. But this present reason is irrational. It is inhumane. It is insupportable.

These are fathers, mothers, children.

They say that one death is worse than one statistic. At least, Joseph Stalin said it this way, meaning it in a certain way, and in this peculiar way he was right.

Millions?

There have been 1.6 million official COVID-deaths to date. A number of these are debatable: Would this one or that person still be alive without COVID? For some of them, the answer is negative; so, should they be counted as COVID-deaths?

On the other hand, many COVID-deaths are not officially counted, out of fear, shame, demoralization, or just a lack of resources. From what I know of this small world, you may count 50% more deaths, uncounted.

Those of you who have read *Minding Corona* know that the worst is yet to come. That is, in 2021, and maybe in 2022, and 2023.

That is the directly COVID-related chunk.

Most deaths will be out of starvation.

In 2021, there will be 270 million people on the brink of starvation, daily, according to the World Food Organization. That is 180 million more than pre-COVID. These are mainly COVID-related due to lockdown, one way or another. Say that only +/- 2% of these will die of hunger and lack of clean water, COVID-related. That easily makes 3.6 million.

With the direct COVID-related death toll in 2021 comparable to 2020, the direct + indirect COVID-related death toll amounts to +/- 6 million.

There's a time when empathy reaches beyond itself.

I'm not talking about sympathy or emotional contagion. [see: "Landscape of Empathy"]

Empathy. You're sitting in a boat, and you don't care anymore. At any moment, you can jump into the water. There is a sea of misery.

Because the horror is so preventable in several ways. For example, the West could act like China.

Daily New Cases in China

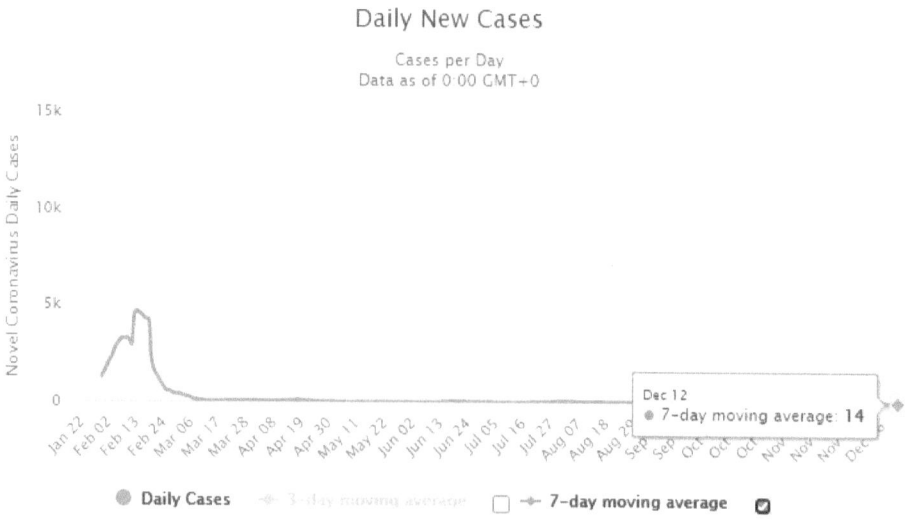

We in the West want our freedom. Goodness. As good as no one in the West knows what freedom is about in the first place. [see: "You Are Free Even While Freedom Is an Illusion"]

The same people don't know what 'I' is about, what consciousness is about, where motivation comes from, what religion is about, what 'human depth' might be, nor even whether rationality might be reasonable after all.

Still, we want 'our freedom.'

In this case, I would prefer China.

Still, the West doesn't need to act like China. Maybe there's value after all in the Western quest for freedom, even while it's misguided at present. It might be a road worth traveling on.

Yeah, it might be a road worth traveling on for China too!

I am convinced. There is strong merit in having the same goal worldwide. People can come together, understand each other, live in peace, and be ready for AI singularity — hopefully, in time.

What a wonderful world (it would be)!

Feet back on the ground. Or, at least, in rationality and science, where we encounter:

Your mind is more powerful than the virus.

Of course.

How powerful? We don't know. My own experiences and scientific wanderings show me that, with optimal support, this may be a matter of millions of lives—saved or squandered. Yes, it is harsh.

Yet today, an extensive search in PubMed reveals almost no attention to this aspect. Remarkably, the few references that I found are by non-Western authors (Iranian, Indian, Chinese). Moreover, they're not of the highest scientific quality.

So, there is little to no experimental science about the influence of the mind on COVID progression, whether positive or negative. There is a ton of theoretical science that shows mind→immune influences. The fact that nowadays, empirical science is necessary to make something 'look like science' is a fleeting historical artifact. There is no intrinsically rational reason for it to be so. It is, in the end, a sociological soon-to-be-relic.

Moreover, in anything mind-health-related, present-day experimental science has already shown to be a fluke. I dare to discuss this with anyone who dares to put his career on the scales. Of course, before he starts putting, I would like to show him the evidence. After that, go ahead, seriously. I mean, 100% seriously.

Vaccination time?

Looking at the present studies, I have this comment:

In a large group of subjects (+/- 30.000), those with heightened vigilance and suggestibility (not gullibility!) may be the first (of the few hundred) to 'feel symptoms' or notice existing minor symptoms, thus being subjectively diagnosed. They may also be the first to break the blind. When sensing to be in the placebo group, they may be feeling/sensing more symptoms (nocebo), thus getting more readily diagnosed. In the mRNA studies, there are several blindness-breakers, such as unblinded administrators. The study may therefore be a measure of vigilance and suggestibility rather than vaccination efficacy.

The clue is that 'placebo' is still not understood well. It is precisely about suggestibility. [see me on PubMed] So, in a novel study design, one can be very wrong — especially with so few subjects in the *real* studies: only a few hundreds. Where in a good double-blind study, the suggestible are rather shunned. Here, not on purpose but by study design, they are distilled from 30.000.

The fact that this has not at all been taken into account is preposterous. We don't know how well the present vaccinations work. My guess is that they will, all in all, probably not influence the death toll much in 2021.

Of course, I know that these deaths form only part of the total misery caused by not wanting to see the true mind-related influence on health and well-being.

It is about so much more.

Yet COVID is new, visible, like the shockwave of a comet hitting the earth from a blue sky.

When I started studying medicine in 1979

I had a vision – I still remember it well – of only getting through seven materialistic years by turning my heart into a stone. I succeeded just enough. Meanwhile, during those years, I did read a lot of literature, poetry, depth psychology, philosophy, and all that really matters for healthcare.

It matters more now than in those years.

Medicine is technical. A good doctor also brings his heart – not just some superficial sympathy – into the consultation room. But that is not medicine. It is the physician as a person.

Medicine itself is technical.

Apart from this, the heart can be brought in different ways. It doesn't even need to be medicine. It may be some kind of mental health hygiene.

Before that happens, millions will keep dying unwarranted deaths from psycho-somatic illness every year. Even more will suffer. Even more than this will not attain their potential.

At least, this deserves our attention.

35. Vaccination Hesitancy: the Good, the Less Good, and the Ugly

December 23, 2020

	Daily	Total
Cases worldwide	683.254	79.036.628
Deaths worldwide	13.468	1.736.720

Preliminaries

This text is also part of a project at ResearchGate: https://www.researchgate.net/project/Minding-Corona]

Before reading this, you may be interested in how to diminish vaccination hesitancy: [see: "How to Make Someone Take His Vaccination"]

The world is about to be vaccinated.

Yet, many people report not wanting the vaccine injected into their bodies. 'Vaccination hesitancy' is a neutral term to denote the latter. I confess that, presently, I am one of the doubters. My hesitancy comes from uncertainty about safety in the long term and effectiveness regarding personal protection as well as herd immunity.

There is a real danger in getting vaccinated if that eventually turns out to be of little use. It may lead to surplus morbidity and mortality. We'll come to that.

We can discern three groups of people who are not keen to get the vaccine.

The distinction is essential for how to (try to) persuade them to get vaccinated if and when appropriate. Making such a distinction is vital to COVID-vaccinations and other vaccinations, as well as other domains of healthcare.

The three groups are:

1. anti-vaxxers

   These get fueled by irrational distrust, spilling over into what others may see as paranoid thinking and behavior. There's a role here for self-enhancement, money, status. However, most anti-vaxxers are just anxious people, comparable to phobic individuals. They are not to be blamed.

   Generally, in this group, there is little respect for rationality. Thus, these people are seldom susceptible to rational arguments. Demonizing a paranoid person doesn't cure him. Quite the opposite: It may strengthen his conviction that "others try to demonize me, so I should be extra cautious and resistant." On the other hand, paranoia doesn't make one unintelligent. Even bright people can be subject to this condition. This way, they can use knowledgeable means to further their cause, attracting followers who additionally heighten the delusion. Not taking this into account would not be intelligent indeed. The situation is real: In the UK, 5.3 million people follow anti-vaxxers accounts on social media, whereas 2.6 million follow the NHS account.

2. wrongfully rational doubters

These are non-experts who follow seemingly rational arguments to their logical conclusions which are clearly wrong to any expert.

These doubters are susceptible to counter-arguments. They put rational arguments in the scale and decide. The solution is straightforward: bring them the correct information.

3. rightfully rational doubters

As even experts can be wrong, and as rational doubt is prominent in any good science, abstractly seen, the last two groups can only be discerned in hindsight. What is right or wrong is to be found in open discussion and communication. The present COVID-vaccinations have a lot to answer for, also regarding their effectiveness. [1][2]

This group is too important to be denied, even though they may dangerously fuel the first group. A correct argumentation may be blown out of proportion. On the other hand, fear of being regarded as an anti-vaxxer might make this group hesitant to come out with rational findings.

Active denial to perceive the third group as a possibility can be another kind of paranoia, cynically realized by people who deem themselves to be utterly rational, thus standing 'above' doubt in their basic conceptions. In many cases, 'rational' stands for 'conceptual' and 'materialistic' in the sense that no place is reserved for subconceptual processing or the non-conscious mind. In view of all the evidence from present-day science, this is delusional. See the burgeoning literature in neurocognitive science.

In such a case, active denial of the subconceptual leads to pseudo-rationality or even anti-rationality.

Disguised as the crux of rationality, this anti-rational stance disconcertingly puts the whole rational effort in dark daylight. This may harden the first group's standpoint: If this is what 'rationality' amounts to, they don't want it, preferring to flush away the whole project of rationality. This way, aggression mounts on both sides. Putting more aggression into it endlessly heightens that of the other side. The result is a mental war zone.

In short, an aggressive stance may make anti-vaxxers more deluded and may make rational doubters more hesitant. It is not indicated towards any of the three groups. This includes verbal aggression in emails and social media, where it's rampant. Open communication is so much better.

Let's look into the title of this piece now:

- *Good* is to be open to a correct argumentation.
- *Best* is to relentlessly strive for a correct argumentation, although good is undoubtedly good enough for most people.
- *Less good* is to be open to rationality but not finding it worthwhile to make some effort for a correct argumentation.
- *Ugly* is any kind of aggression. At present, there's a lot of aggression towards the first group. There is also a lot of aggression coming from the first group. From their point of view, it's understandable. Much pent-up energy (deep motivation) shows itself this way, resulting in a kind of radicalization.

We should not promote the vaccines beyond any doubt *just because* "people would otherwise be more hesitant." That would be an ill-advised attempt to motivate the masses, actually coming down to manipulation — guaranteed to result in much resistance. Only a scientifically open attitude is serious and respectful, thus mandatory. Moreover, if vaccines after some time would not appear to work for > 50%, we would face meanwhile

dire consequences:

- A huge financial cost is to be weighed against a less positive impact.
- Many people's side effects, even some mortality, are also to be weighed against a less positive impact.
- Corona-tired people get increasingly demotivated to use other protection measures after being vaccinated with what they think to be highly protective.
- The search for more valid COVID therapies becomes less urgent.
- The search for better vaccines becomes unjustifiably hampered, for instance, through subjects in the placebo groups of trials not willing to forego vaccination by the seemingly very potent ones.
- People who get ill despite vaccination (showing gradually over months) are additionally blamed for being too careless — as they will be, especially those who need to be careless to get food on the table.
- If it becomes apparent that the vaccines are much less effective, many may lose faith in vaccines, and perhaps in science generally. The Anti-vax movement gets more vigorous. We will have a hard time distributing even better-working vaccines.
- The virus may become vaccine-resistant, like bacteria becoming antibiotics-resistant when antibiotics are carelessly used en masse in suboptimal doses. Only, the virus may appear to mutate quicker, thus also growing resistance quicker.

Let's go deeper into the last point, shifting a bit from the central subject of this text, but as an example of it. Note the difference between viral shift (one big change) and viral drift (many small changes). Note also that I'm not a virologist. But due to the complexity of immunology and vaccinology, and the situation's novelty, we should seriously take this into account. For sure, we have never before witnessed the present situation: mass vaccination against a relatively quickly mutating organism. For instance, the scale of vaccination against Influenza is much smaller.

So, if the vaccine works for, say, only 50%, then each time a person gets ill and infective despite vaccination, the virus within that person may have learned to overcome the vaccine-immune shield against it. This more resistant virus may mean a further drift towards a 'vaccine-resistant strain.' Through the mass scaling, vaccine-resistance by the virus may build up with special vigor. The consequence is that through the vaccination itself, we boost the virus to mutate beyond it. We attack the enemy, and the enemy defends itself.

The principle: This kind of vaccination engenders mutation and resistance.

This principle may also be relevant to Influenza vaccinations. Drifting viruses jump all over the connected world onboard humans in airplanes. Viral resistance may build up in developed, vaccinated areas, then incubate further in underdeveloped, underfed, non-vaccinated areas. After a while, we see that "a new resistant strain comes from the East this year." But mutation and incubation do not need to happen at the same spot. This may also take place with coronaviruses.

The result: Rich people getting vaccinated repeatedly with accommodated vaccines. Before the new vaccines reach poor people, the virus has mainly grown beyond, and the cycle repeats itself in wave after wave. The rich keep themselves vaccinated and relatively safe. *Through* their self-vaccination, the virus mutates quicker and wreaks havoc with the poor. If this comes to be, I hope it will be managed with Compassion.

A possible scenario with disappointing results of vaccinations

may be met by confounding 'reasons' for this:

- "It is wintertime, in which the virus appears to be more virulent."
- "The virus has significantly mutated, meanwhile. There are many new strains."
- "Those who are vaccinated are more careless and thus get more infected. The vaccine works well, but people's behavior is counteracting."

- "It is a mystery. We don't know what is happening. This virus behaves in many weird ways."
- "It is a coincidence and a combination of all these factors."

In such case, the reaction might lie in not doubting the vaccine studies but in striving to reach 'more of the same': new developments, new vaccinations, additional money-flow to those companies who are already on the market, and prolongation of immense, unnecessary suffering.

Where is the human mind in all this?

Nothing is straightforward.

With the present evidence, one can be wrong in both directions, denying what is or promoting what is not. In retrospect, it will be challenging to appreciate the other side. In any case, one should not blame anyone as long as the intentions are sincere.

However, one way to avoid much suffering is by demanding from the industry the use of treatment assumptions, thus making the blindness of double-blind studies more what it is supposed to be, enhancing the joint scientific effort towards better healthcare and, eventually, people's health and well-being. [3] [4] [see also: "Double-Blind in the Balance"]

[1]   https://blogs.bmj.com/bmj/2020/11/26/peter-doshi-pfizer-and-modernas-95-effective-vaccines-lets-be-cautious-and-first-see-the-full-data/

[2] https://www.bmj.com/content/371/bmj.m4924/rr-0 (note, as author, your humble author)

[3] https://www.researchgate.net/publication/347511352 The Importance of Testing for Blindness in COVID-19 Vaccination Trials

[4] https://www.researchgate.net/publication/347841803 Serial Treatment

Assumption Testing STAT Towards Better Evidence for Evidence Based
 Medicine

36. Vaccine or Vaccination?

This text is not for the faint-hearted. Even so, before you read on, make sure you understand that MUCH OF THIS IS STILL HYPOTHETICAL, HOWEVER, PROBABLE ENOUGH TO BE TAKEN INTO ACCOUNT.

February 6, 2021

	Daily	Total
Cases worldwide	495.819	105.906.560
Deaths worldwide	14.592	2.307.879

Please, in any case, read this

It's not because psychotherapy works (very well, even) that psychotherapeutic models and techniques work. With scientific certainty, they don't. [see: "The Case Against Psychotherapies"]

It's not because 650.000 knee operations of a specific kind were performed in the US annually with good results that the procedure itself was effective. It wasn't. [see: "A Tale of Placebo: Arthritis of the Knee"]

It's not because some 250 million people take antidepressants daily that these work very well apart from placebo. According to the type of study, their placebo-part ranges from 80% to nearly 100%.

Etc. etc.

Before you laugh away the following, you should have proper answers to many issues such as those above or at least one excellent depthless answer to one of them. Spoiler alert: there is none.

So:

It's not because COVID-vaccinations (in broad context) work well that COVID-vaccines work well.

You remember my image of the whirlpool in which material and mental factors play a role. Imagine being near the whirlpool. A few steps in one or the other direction are enough to keep safe or not. That's all it needs — not much. According to one hypothesis, apparently, the vaccination is enough to perform this for the time being.

According to the same hypothesis, humanity is soon made to fly on only one decently acknowledged wing. If, for one reason or the other (many candidates exist), faith in the other wing evaporates, it doesn't work anymore, and people may fall in droves.

I cannot readily think of a more dangerous situation in the history of humankind. At least, with science in mind and with what is at stake, it should be investigated. It should have been a year ago.

I send this message to the future: I did my best. Before you judge me, please take into account the whole situation. My name is Jean-Luc, not Lucky Luke the Lonesome Cowboy, although I can shoot pretty well if need be.

Curves and numbers

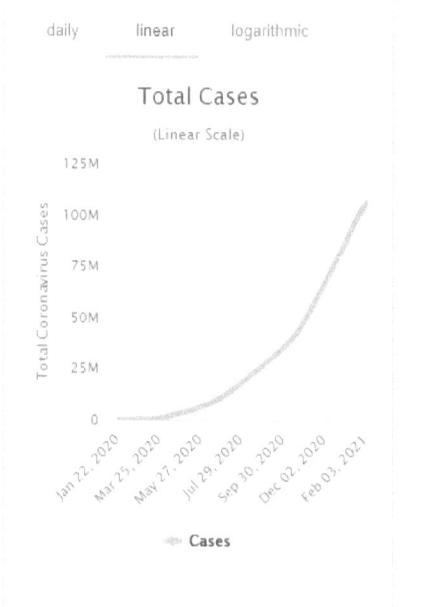 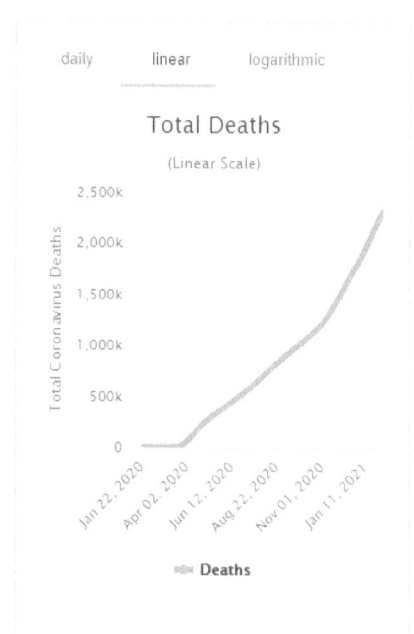

(from https://www.worldometers.info/coronavirus/)

There is some slowing down in these numbers, worldwide, hesitatingly, while the hope of many rests on the shoulders of vaccines. Massive campaigns are put in place to get as many people vaccinated as possible.

The quickest progress is made in Israel, with one-third of the population already vaccinated. Reports show excellent results in numbers of cases of infection and deaths (effectiveness is up to > 90%). The differences between the vaccinated and the non-vaccinated are remarkable. A point of caution is that this comes during a tightening of the third Israeli lockdown. As to mortality in the total Israeli population, this is the curve today from https://www.worldometers.info/coronavirus/country/israel/:

Daily New Deaths in Israel

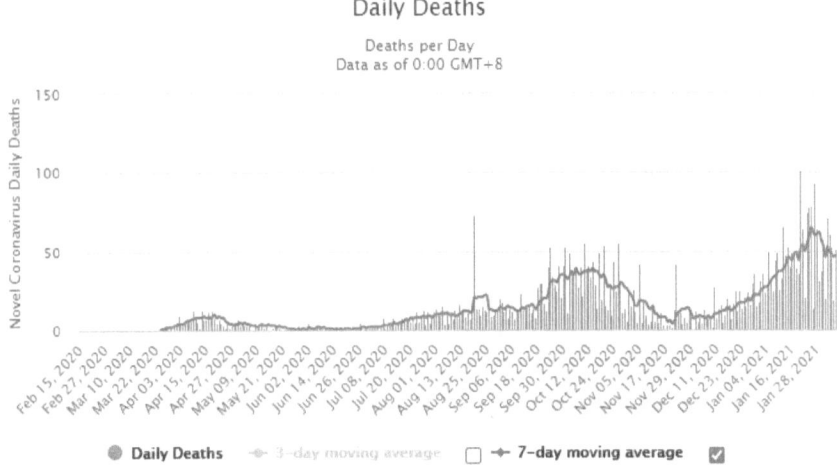

Daily Deaths

Deaths per Day
Data as of 0:00 GMT+8

Does this show the effect of the vaccines?

Several vaccine RCTs have revealed a high to very high efficacy. However, scrutinizing this research in light of placebo, nocebo, and blindness breach, the results of the studies may be seriously flawed. This means, they are inconclusive. I posted some rapid responses about this in the British Medical Journal:

- https://www.bmj.com/content/371/bmj.m4924/rr-0
- https://www.bmj.com/content/371/bmj.m4924/rr-5
- https://www.bmj.com/content/371/bmj.m4924/rr-6

These are not very uplifting.

Note that this is what science is supposed to be about: being critical. Different opinions need to be put beside each other. Ignoring something because the mind is – or is not – involved is preposterous and, in this case, dangerous.

Science is <u>not</u> just being critical up to where it doesn't suit one anymore. Science doesn't stop at the exit where money and status might be lost. It goes on and on. This eternal doubt and tenacity are why science is our only hope. If it is taken away, humanity is pretty lost. We need more science. Also, we need better science. This endeavor should never end.

Stress virus?

As you may have read in my book, COVID is more than simply a viral disease. As a matter of fact, virus is virus. The COVID disease is caused not by the virus but by a combination of factors in which the immune system and stress also play important roles. This combination forms a whirlpool in which people can get caught when making unfortunate moves at crucial times.

Of course, we're not getting anywhere by looking at stress as an amorphous blob that inhabits one like some chemical element. Stress is about meaning. [see: "Not Stress but Meaning is a Cause of Disease."] Thus, it is about striving for autonomy and life itself. [see: "The Autonomy and the Meaning"]

Social nocebo

In another article [see on RG: "The Role of Social Nocebo in COVID-19"], I expanded on 'mass psychogenic illness:' symptoms or illness that may befall many people in a joint happening that can also be seen as a whirlpool. This is a social whirlpool. It seems to happen regularly but is seldom reported. In many cases, there is shame or avoidance of guilt involved, and a covering it up with some somatic cloak, or just ignoring and forgetting it.

This is one of the reasons why I prefer the term 'social nocebo:' less negative connotation. Another reason is that it brings the happening closer to a domain of which much is already known: true placebo phenomena.

Vaccination

With 'vaccination,' I denote the whole bio-psycho-social context in which the vaccine-as-product is administered. Lending hope and positive expectation to many may diminish the power of social nocebo. This diminishment of nocebo may also be seen as a placebo. Opening the concept this way, we may look for insight in the literature about placebo.

There's a lot. Placebo is real and robust.

This is not about other vaccines. In my view, COVID is special in its stress-relatedness, in the appearance and disappearance of a COVID-whirlpool. Nevertheless, the principle of a whirlpool may be relevant to many other psycho-somatic illnesses.

Bringing it all together

My apprehension about effectiveness of the COVID vaccine is considerable. Note that I am no anti-vaxxer [see: "Vaccination Hesitancy: the Good, the less Good, and the Ugly"]. But, as said, good science doesn't stop quickly.

There may be much placebo involved in the vaccine studies, especially in the age ranges where it matters most. With little data – being all we've got in these studies – and thus with huge uncertainty, I calculate a placebo-effect of +/- 80% concerning severe COVID cases in the Pfizer study. [see on RG: "Efficacy of placebo-vaccine administration on occurrences of severe COVID-19"]

Note also that in this study, people were blinded as to receiving a vaccine versus a placebo. In the real world, there is no blindness. People know they get the vaccine. Thus, the placebo effect may be higher.

One may ask whether any placebo can be so powerful.

The short answer is: yes. [see: "How Active is Placebo?"] A side-note to this: We know little about the placebo of vaccinations. We know more about the placebo of medications and increasingly more about medical procedures, including operations. In any of these, studies occasionally show huge effects.

Like: more placebo than pharmaco.

20%? 40%? 80%?

In the case of COVID vaccination, we don't know. Proper studies to find out have not been done. If the placebo-effect of the COVID vaccination is substantial, then we are at risk of floating on a placebo cloud, massively. In that case, the situation may be much more dangerous than that of antidepressants.

What if the cloud bursts? With medication, such a burst is rather individual. With vaccination, it is rather social, with problems way more difficult to contain.

I have written about this in "Why it Matters to Know the Real Effectiveness."

There is reason to be cautious. It is not a question of 'freedom or no freedom.' A division in two opposing camps 'for versus against lockdown' doesn't make sense to me. It hinders both parties in trying to reach a good global picture to be reached as a stable equilibrium. It leads to a labile equilibrium in which the strongest party wins, creating much stress near a lurching whirlpool.

That should be avoided.

As said, this is all hypothetical

as is also the basis upon which the mass vaccinations are being rolled out.

If the hypothesis of this text is correct, I see two main consequences:

- The vaccinations are making the situation extremely, insanely dangerous. Namely: Many people do not understand the 'power of placebo,' equating it with sheer make-belief and deception. While, of course, placebo is deception – one way or another – the 'power of placebo' is far from it. If the placebo-deception gets punctured, it may deflate into nothing or may even flip-flop towards a social nocebo phenomenon. The real strength of the second wing lies in the 'power of placebo,' not in the placebo itself.

- Much more attention should go to the mind as a causal factor (thus, also important towards management). One can do so socially and individually. This is not to say that it would be unimportant in the other case. The lack of attention to ourselves is mind-boggling anyway.

Things are not black or white.

If the vaccination placebo is vast, it points to a way – within ourselves – to alleviate the present problems enormously, rashly, with little cost, little need for lockdown, and more positive outcomes than merely COVID-related.

This is about being fully human. The main question then would be: Do we dare?

ADDENDUM

February 21, 2021

	Daily	Total
Cases worldwide	372.498	111.638.837
Deaths worldwide	8.493	2.471.484

Since mid-January 2021, worldwide cases are dropping markedly. Two weeks later, also mortality. This trend is continuing. It is not a glitch.

Why are COVID-19 cases dropping fast?

Several reasons have been put forward:

1. behavior change: people worldwide have finally got the hang of wearing masks and social distancing
2. seasonality: winter months being corona months
3. partial immunity: many people having been infected, thus immunized naturally
4. vaccines/vaccinations

Personally, at present, I don't believe in 1 since I see no reason for it. It seems to be just any explanation after the facts, something in which humans excel (including me).

Also, I don't believe in 2. If anything, seasonality should be moving us in the opposite direction.

A substantial factor may be 3.

About 4, we don't know how much, but the vaccines by themselves probably contribute. Note that the reduction of cases began _before_ the vaccinations started being rolled out.

Where is 5: the mind in all this? Where can it be? One can only hypothesize. A seemingly good explanation to me is the mindset brought about by the vaccinations' success in studies and media. A good job has been done in pushing this. The social nocebo spell may have been taken away by bringing hope that the end of the tunnel may be approaching.

In conclusion, factors 3, 4, and 5 may be taking energy out of the COVID whirlpool. Which factor is most important?

Of course, the dropping in cases is super. Also, we should definitely continue with the vaccinations.

Still, for obvious reasons and more, it is crucial to know what really happened, is happening, and will probably happen. Most of all, we urgently need to know who we are. The viral threat is still present. The next threats will be with us soon enough.

37. 1.5 Years of Mindless COVID

Boring news: We still don't know much directly about the influence of the mind on COVID, nor about the placebo effect of COVID vaccinations. The world of science is unfathomably silent.

June 5, 2021

	Daily	Total
Cases worldwide	475.717	172.894.435
Deaths worldwide	10.737	3.716.853

This time of the year, as last year, in Belgium, the atmosphere is one of 'huge relief after doing the right thing.' This time around, the vaccinations are part of the exuberance. We're out of the woods!

I genuinely hope so... mostly. Let's compare the numbers.

7-day average COVID deaths at the 3rd of June

Last year compared to this:

	2020	2021
Belgium	23	13
Worldwide	5.043	10.271

Is this positive or negative?

Noteworthy, going one year back and five days forward in Belgium, we were at 13 deaths per day. That's the same as today. Does this say anything with certainty? Hmm.

Taking a few other European countries, same day of same month, 7-day averages:

	2020	2021
Italy	78	78
Spain	31	30
Germany	24	130
Netherlands	12	10
France	58	71

A lot has happened over the year. Second waves. Third waves. Despairs following reliefs after despairs. Worldwide, millions have died. And, of course: the vaccinations.

I remember that last year, the drop around this time of the year came as a surprise. This year, same thing. That is not a good sign. To me, it's worrying since it fits in a dangerous scheme. [see: "COVID Whirlpool"]

What is the placebo effect of COVID vaccinations? What is the total impact of the mind on COVID? Where would we be without vaccinations? Where would we be with a proper use of specific mind-related interventions?

These are difficult questions.

Whoever knows the answer is a fool.

Including me. I don't know the answers. I can only guess after trying to get the most relevant facts together.

Like everybody else, I can see that after the vaccination campaigns – in countries doing well on these – numbers of deaths have dropped dramatically. That is excellent!

But what is the cause?

Let's look at the data from some other countries, 7-day averages:

	2020	2021
US	997	390
UK	173	11
Israel	1	3
Mexico	624	96

Brazil	1.492	1.862
China	0	0
Japan	7	92
India	275	2.706
Lithuania	0	9
Hungary	4	20
Argentina	38	534
Colombia	38	523

This doesn't prove to me that the vaccines don't work. These numbers also do not prove they work. Much depends on circumstantial factors. Mainly: how well do people comply with viral hygiene?

And of course: how does the mind fit in? What comes with hope – or, on the other side, despair – in the mind frames of many people concerning COVID and other factors?

The hope through the vaccinations themselves has been built up with immense power.

Also, can there be a 'regression to the mean' involved in, for instance, Mexico? Simply, after a big surge, one can expect a big drop. This happens frequently in medicine with many diseases. In Mexico, with a vaccination degree of 13% at this time, the search is on for an explanation of the huge drop. What researchers come up with is tentative (compliance, season, good luck, herd immunity, proximity to the US). It looks to me like 'anything goes.'

My tentative explanation: With regression to the mean, the COVID whirlpool gets relaxed, leading to a drop that is (much) bigger than expected.

Let's hope my tentative explanation is not correct.

Looking at vaccinated people

[From: "Effectiveness of Pfizer-BioNTech and Moderna Vaccines Against COVID-19 Among Hospitalized Adults Aged ≥65 Years - United States, January-March 2021" https://pubmed.ncbi.nlm.nih.gov/33956782/]

Among 417 hospitalized adults aged ≥65 years (including 187 case-patients and 230 controls), this shows vaccination effectiveness of 94% after full vaccination. The 95%-confidence interval (49%-99%) is huge, bringing its own uncertainty, but let's say the success of vaccination is 94%. Does this prove that the vaccines are very effective or that the placebo effect of getting the vaccines is huge? In theory, both are possible. [see: "Vaccine or Vaccination?"]

The more you would know about placebo, the more you would find it likely.

But the initial big studies?

Following this last link, you find some other links to posted – by me – rapid answers in the *British Medical Journal* concerning the initial vaccine studies. These are far from evidently straightforward. The placebo concept has been mismanaged thoroughly.

Of course, to not-know is not the same as to know-that-not.

At present, we know little. Even the vaccine-induced antibodies in the blood bring no certitude. It is a very complex domain, in which I am no expert, but I can read what other experts say in openness. All good science depends on the latter.

But placebo – worldwide – so many people—seriously?

That's probably the main question. Is this at all possible?

If the question is whether so many domain experts can look right through it without seeing it, then that is certainly possible. I've had more than my share of practical experience regarding COVID and other healthcare issues.

Many weirder things have been debunked in the history of humankind. For instance, the history of medicine has been termed the 'history of placebo' by top-level researchers in the domain, with many thousands of different pills and potions etc. that all were popular some day and since have been unveiled as 100% placebos. The least one can say is that people are prone to this. [*The powerful placebo: From ancient priest to modern physician*, 1997]

Even now, the placebo plays a much heavier role in entire Western healthcare than most people imagine. [see: "Studies Show: Placebos as

Effective as Treatment"] I don't see it being different in other parts of the world.

Placebo/nocebo

It's challenging to compare the placebo effect of medication to that of vaccination — especially as we are witnessing now at a grand scale.

In both cases, the placebo can also be seen as a diminishment of social nocebo. Still, in mass vaccinations, probably more. This can play an immense role in the present conundrum. [see RG: "The Role of Social Nocebo in COVID-19"]

This depends on the mind's influence in the first place. Therefore, it should not be transposed to many other vaccinations, which are certainly very efficient.

COVID is different. Lots of elements point to the influence of the mind-brain, in this case, the COVID whirlpool. [see: "COVID Whirlpool"]

The COVID future is still uncertain.

Worrisome: seasonality, viral shifts (variants), an almost certain drop in vaccine efficiency, the non-global reach of vaccination campaigns, demotivated people, long-term side effects of vaccinations, 'long haulers' (people keeping symptoms) after infection.

Hopeful: development of vaccines that work increasingly well —keeping up with variants, the effect of herd immunity.

Winter in America (and Europe), cold again?

Hypothetically, next winter in the West, we will see a new substantial COVID wave in which the mind will play a crucial role — again. As usual, the mind will be discarded, and thus, so will its influence in the COVID whirlpool.

Meanwhile, the virus keeps on shifting and drifting with certainty. Of course, not seeing the mind, 'new variants' can be put forward as the cause of the wave(s). This will definitely be possible and backed up by laboratory data, but not, therefore, most sensible or correct. Data may be accurate and excruciatingly incomplete. As I see it, this is 'the history of scientific medicine.'

Not the science is wrong, but the scientists, time and again, concerning the mind.

I started a research group on ResearchGate months ago.

This had little success until now. [see RG: "Minding Corona"]

If you are a researcher, you can join. The intention is to foster scientific research concerning mind-influences on COVID. With a group of ten, we can go for it. The free-for-always app that I developed one year ago (April 2020) can be used in this research. [see: "Free App to Relieve COVID"]

Still worthwhile +++

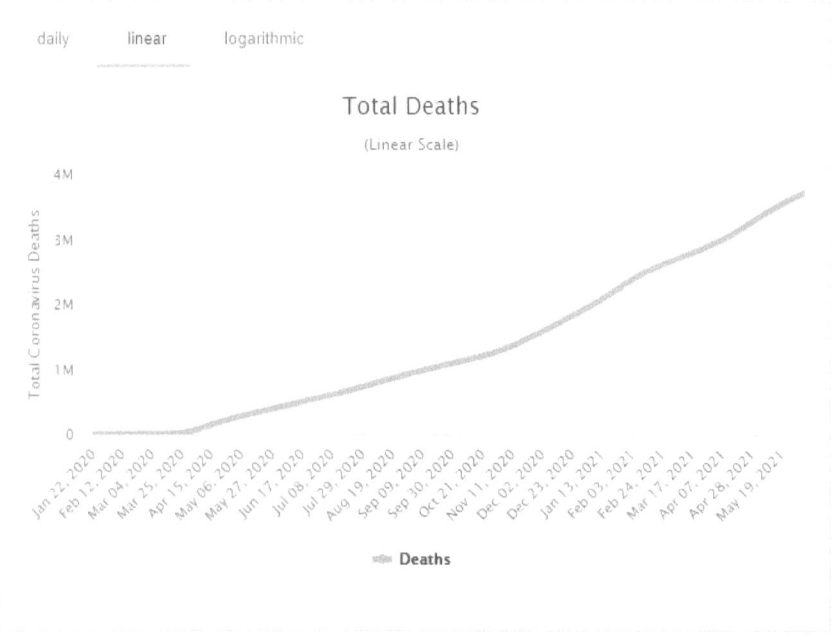

Looking at the above numbers and this graph (from https://www.worldometers.info/coronavirus/), the world is still very much under the spell of COVID. Also, even in vaccinated countries, there is the continual threat of terrible variants. The more new infections, the higher the chances. Remember that it probably all started with one infection.

Minding the mind will always remain vital in COVID.

Also, looking at the post-COVID future, we should keep going.

We, human beings, are much more interesting than we pretend to be, even though individuals – in their superficiality, NOT as total persons – may be the subject or object of dislike.

If we don't learn the lesson, the future is very bleak.

38. Winter of 2021: COVID Winter AGAIN!?

Some evolutions worry me into thinking that next winter will be a hard one again, in which the COVID whirlpool will again be relevant in Europe, certainly worldwide.

July 5, 2021

	Daily	Total
Cases worldwide	344.785	184,932,708
Deaths worldwide	6.275	4,000,675

[see: "COVID-Whirlpool - In Which Virus AND Mind Play Substantial Roles"]

COVID-19 is a psycho-somatic disease.

I'm sorry to have to say this: The virus-related experts everybody listens to are somatic. Since it is a psycho-somatic disease, these are the wrong experts, from the start onwards.

Of course, virologists etc. are needed. Even more needed are psycho-somatic experts.

Viral shift versus drift

Every virus, seen as the whole of individual viral elements of that species, evolves continuously in the sense of minor changes as well as bigger ones. These can be seen as steps and jumps. The difference is quite arbitrary. New viral variants are mostly the results of jumps. At present, for instance, Western Europe sees the rise of the delta-variant.

Through steps and jumps, the virus eventually becomes so much changed that specific vaccinations lose their power. The immune system doesn't recognize the virus anymore. Gradually, we need a new vaccination.

The more steps the virus takes, the smaller the jump needed to reach this stage. Also, the more the virus gets dispersed, the easier it finds its way towards change in the direction of higher infectiousness and vaccine-resistance.

End result: We will see more variants evolving towards vaccine-resistance at a quicker than expected pace.

The genie in the vaccine

How big is the placebo-factor of COVID-vaccinations? I've delved into this question before. [see: "Vaccine or Vaccination?"]

Placebo comes as a factor of pattern recognition and completion. [see: "Placebo and the Predictive Brain"] Part of the pattern is the viral element as recognized by the immune system. Mental elements form another part. The whole is like a genie in a bottle that appears when the bottle is treated in a certain way.

If the bottle itself changes, the genie appears less easily, impacting the turning of the whirlpool.

End result: The placebo-factor of COVID-vaccinations may diminish in a non-linear way, thus also the power of vaccinations, quicker than expected. This depends on the height of the placebo-effect, of which at present, we know little to nothing.

One can foresee in both cases that the quicker-than-expected pace plays a higher role in developing countries/regions with lower vaccination grades to start with. New variants will mainly come from these regions.

Big Pharma is not to blame,

let alone the people working there.

With one remark on this: They should keep thinking, also out of the viral box. They may say this is not their job. Well, who's job is it? Please tell me!

Still waging war

We're waging war where we shouldn't because, within that war, we ourselves are part of what we are waging it against.

The war that is waged here is one exponent of what is happening in many fields, although in a hidden way. It's a war inside. [see: "The Battle of the Future"]

When are we going to transcend this?

What is needed to open your eyes, Prof. Braeckman, Prof. Benedetti, and so many others?

39. What if COVID Vaccinations are 80% Placebo?

This question still needs to be asked given the probability, lack of disproof, and immensity of the consequences.

July 25, 2021

	Daily	Total
Cases worldwide	492.082	194,374,131
Deaths worldwide	8.299	4.168.100

I want as many people as possible to get vaccinated.

I'm the opposite of an anti-vaxxer. [see: "How to Make Someone Take His Vaccination"]

We need good science, as much as possible. This requires good rationality. This requires a good view of reality. In reality, there is no choice as to what one perchance wants or does not want to see — including the deeper aspects of the human mind. [see: "The Basic Cognitive Illusion"]

Surprisingly?

Also, to me, 80% would be surprisingly high, but not unimaginable. We've seen comparable things in the history of medicine.

I use the image of a whirlpool in which virus- and mind-related factors enhance each other. [see: "COVID-Whirlpool"] Thus, the virus may be 100% needed, and still, mind-related factors may also be needed to get the morbid or even deadly whirlpool going. The vaccine's placebogenic help to drop the mind factors to below a threshold may be enough. The 'placebo' may in this case also be thought of as a diminishment of nocebo. One can think of it as taking a few steps towards inside or outside a whirlpool. Not much is needed for a huge difference. For several reasons, it's still important to know what is really happening. [see: "Why It Matters to Know the Real Effectiveness."] It is unfathomable to me to see the absence of research, and even the active denial of researchers in this. I just do not get it. Additionally, there is general denial by the population globally. This doesn't show the power of (dis)belief. That has been shown by other research well enough. But it sure shows the amount of (dis)believers. Multiplicate and be surprised of nothing.

Logically, if you have more than one +/- necessary condition to a consequence, and you take out any of them, the consequence is +/- not reached anymore. In COVID, young age is such a condition. In my view, mind-related factors ('stress') are another one. Of course, 'stress' as a category is much too blunt. [see: "Not Stress but Meaning Is a Cause of Disease."] Note that since the start, practically no experimental research has been done regarding the causal influence of the mind on COVID progression. The few small studies that I know of were positive.

COVID may be pretty much a psycho-somatic disease, with the mind playing a causal role in COVID progression to an as yet unknown degree. [see: "The Role of Social Nocebo in COVID-19"] Circumstantial evidence tells a story with virus *and* mind at the center. I urge everybody to take this seriously. [see: "Minding COVID: a Different Story"]

About placebo and nocebo

It's not entirely correct to speak exclusively about the placebo effect of a vaccine. It's possibly as much about the diminishment of nocebo through feeling the safety of being vaccinated. [see: "Is Social Nocebo Real?"] These concepts have fuzzy borders. For the sake of easiness, I keep talking about placebo in this text.

Suppose there is an 80% placebo effect of vaccination. Even so, there would be a 20% effect of the 'naked' vaccine. More importantly, the 80% placebo would need the vaccine itself to be realized.

If you, dear reader, would think that we would just need to grab the placebo effect and leave the vaccine in the bottle, I would advise you to think some more. It's by far not that simple.

7-day average COVID deaths on the 24th of July

I did the same exercise as on the 3rd of June 2021, comparing last year to this, and coming to the same overall picture:

	2020	2021
Belgium	2	1
Worldwide	6.207	8.109

Is this positive or negative? In my view, we're not where we want to be. There's still a huge need to use every available instrument, even ourselves.

Again, taking a few other European countries, the same day of the same month, 7-day averages:

	2020	2021
Italy	8	12
Spain	2	15
Germany	6	20
Netherlands	1	3
France	9	21

These countries + Belgium together:

together:	28	72

As you can see, there were 2.5 x more deaths yesterday (7-day average) than precisely a year ago. Meanwhile, in all these countries, vaccinations are fully on their way.

So is the delta-variant, and so are other variants that we don't yet know. Several may be brooding in remote places or even in Europe. The more we whirl around geographically, the better the virus likes it.

Of course, most of the mortality happens in the group of non-vaccinated people. The issue is not with this but with what is happening under the hood.

Let's look at the data from some other countries (the same list on the 3rd of June), 7-day averages:

	2020	2021
US	952	252
UK	10	64
Israel	8	1
Mexico	777	297
Brazil	1.097	1.105
China	0	0
Japan	1	12
India	388	478
Lithuania	0	1
Hungary	0	1
Argentina	197	311
Colombia	250	366

In the US, the situation is much better now than a year ago. The whole world remembers the mental turmoil of last year, the politicization, the panic and despair. I dare say these may have been crucial factors. This accords well with the minding-corona hypothesis.

What also strikes me are the huge ups and downs in individual countries. There may be several explanations for this. One of them is a whirlpool phenomenon in which the mind plays a substantial role.

About the adversary

Looking at the virus as a conglomerate of all viral particles globally, we have a flexible 'adversary.' It continually changes. Its tentacles (variants) constantly spread in many directions. Its one goal is to be successful as a conglomerate, which one can see as an organism in its own right.

Its 'thinking' is done through sheer trial and error. It doesn't want to kill us. It wants to use us. We're its fertile ground. If it kills us all, it will also disappear. Unfortunately, 'trial and error' isn't an ingenious strategy. This means that a far deadlier version may be on its way. Many scientists were already expecting this before COVID. It's one more reason to take our mind-related resources seriously and try to make the most of it, not only for the sake of now.

From the standpoint of the virus, its strategy is efficient enough for the time being. Its main thrust seems to lie in speed and flexibility, tricking our psycho-neuro-immune system while not looking back in searching for new ground. This makes us vulnerable in specific ways and possibly for a long time.

The huge initial COVID studies

I still see and hear experts talk about the Pfizer & Moderna studies (total 65.000 subjects) and others as double-blind mega-studies showing huge efficacy. This is wrong in the following sense:

- The mega-studies were about adverse reactions. Well done.
- Only +/- 340 people got COVID-diagnosed in the Pfizer & Moderna studies. This number was set beforehand. These 340 were the ones on which the comparison was made between vaccinated and non-vaccinated subjects. So, the efficacy study was done on a mediocre number of subjects. Concerning efficacy, these were not mega-studies.

Moreover, as I described in some BMJ responses, these studies were substantially flawed (see references). The double-blind quality was meager, and an inadvertent placebo-proneness may have significantly skewed the results. [see: "COVID Vaccination Studies: From Double-Blind to Hardly-Blind?"]

The public vaccination results

As described in [see: "Vaccine or Vaccination?"], the scale of the happenings is no guarantee that the supposed hypothesis is correct. I mentioned a few examples. The most interesting function of science – including medical – is to ensure that common-sense suppositions are not false.

Compare it to a stage magician. Many people, including M.D.s and Ph.D.s, may be in the audience. The magician pulls a rabbit out of his hat. Wow! How did he do this? Nobody sees how. So, is he a real magician? Of course not! Yet, the rabbit is real.

Back to COVID vaccinations. The results are real and visible to anybody. But they do not prove the cause. So, where is the causal thinking that also takes the mind into account? It is nowhere.

Also, depending on the type of virus, the science on the efficiency of vaccinations isn't all that straightforward, as shown by a Cochrane report on influenza. [see: "MINDING CORONA, Saving Livelihoods and Lives"]

What we need is good science as much as possible, especially now. This is more than the one that makes us comfortable in desirable suppositions.

But… so many people?

Can all these people be subject to the placebo effect?

Sure. All you need for this is a brain (and body). Placebo is related to a natural characteristic of how the brain works not only in special circumstances but all the time. [see: "Placebo and the Predictive Brain"]

Research on suggestiveness also shows that almost everyone is prone to the placebo effect with enough flexibility in how it is brought. Moreover, in the case of COVID vaccinations, we have several characteristics that specifically enhance their placebogenic power, such as:

- The placebo effect of injections is notably more significant than that of pills.
- The more people involved, the bigger the placebo effect. Here, the whole world is involved.
- We see huge 'marketing' efforts towards making people be vaccinated.

- The initial studies keep being projected as massive studies proving the efficacy.
- Most people are (very) eager to get the shots as lifesavers.
- Many people have to wait a considerable time for their shots.
- People see that massive efforts are being done to get the shots at the right place.
- Nobody talks about a possible placebo effect.
- Much weight is given to the idea of 'This is a triumph of science.' I still hope it will be.

Mind-stuff

A placebo effect of 80% would mean that the mind is a powerful instrument if we can make good use of it. This text by itself does not indicate how important mind-stuff is.

We could have investigated it in conjunction with the vaccination studies. Understandably, there was no interest in this. The pharmaceutical companies wanted to build their case.

At present, performing double-blinded vaccination studies with additional arms to investigate the placebo part is not feasible.

AURELIS app

This app contains information and many mental exercises. [see: "Free App to Relieve COVID"] I developed it last year specifically towards COVID (while also valuable for other fields). It is free, forever. If you think this is 'commercial,' please tell me what to do differently.

This app can be used straightforwardly in studies to investigate the efficacy and effectiveness of the app while at the same time also the influence of the mind on COVID progression — what should have been done already a year ago. It can be used preventively inside and outside of hospitals. Double-blind studies are not possible. Also, they are less needed since a placebo arm would basically just show more influence from the mind. This stands open to argumentation as part of the study. After the study, the same app can be implemented on a vast scale.

Positive results would show the influence of the mind on COVID-progression, possibly also infectiousness. Let's not dwell on what could have been. It only breaks my heart. If positive to very positive, there would be severe consequences towards the future, such as:

- New variants may break through vaccinations more quickly.
- People who don't want to be vaccinated may better protect themselves (and others).
- Protection may be brought where there is no money for mass vaccinations.
- It's low cost. Even better, it's +/- no cost.
- It may be an opening to psycho-somatic insights and implementation in many fields.
- It may bring the importance of empathy and Compassion into medical science.

Brexit?

Serendipitously,   I   read today: https://www.brusselstimes.com/news/belgium-all-news/health/178864/research-how-a-new-covid-variant-sows-its-seeds/

> "The study, the largest of its kind, looked at the alpha variant of the virus, previously known as the Kent or British variant. At one time it was thought that the variant was 80% more transmissible than the standard virus, which accounted for its rapid spread. But the new study shows that is not true. In fact, the alpha variant spread by a succession of 'super-seeder' events."

These new data are compatible with my 'Brexit Stress' rapid response to BMJ of December: https://www.bmj.com/content/371/bmj.m4944/rr-1 . After all, the main problem was not the much higher transmissibility. Moreover, put 'stress' as a super seeder engine in the events, and you're there.

Meanwhile, I'm worried about the theta-plus-variant.

Rest assured. That one doesn't exist yet, except in my nightmare. But with the numbers of today and the mind-boggling negligence of the human species, the viral organism may get there soon enough.

Note that the delta-variant appears to be somewhat more vaccine-resistant. The theta-plus-variant may be pretty vaccine-resistant and adapted to youth. From the virus's standpoint, both would be obvious win situations.

Need I make some drawings?

Meanwhile, in the news already [https://www.npr.org/sections/health-shots/2021/07/22/1019475669/delta-variant-will-drive-a-steep-rise-in-covid-deaths-model-shows]:

> "The current COVID-19 surge in the U.S.—fueled by the **highly contagious delta variant**—will steadily accelerate through the summer and fall, peaking in mid-October, with daily deaths more than triple what they are now. ... It's a deflating prospect for parents looking ahead to the coming school year, employers planning to get people back to the workplace and everyone hoping that the days of big national surges were over."

I fear even this is optimistic.

References

- https://www.bmj.com/content/371/bmj.m4924/rr-0
- https://www.bmj.com/content/371/bmj.m4924/rr-5
- https://www.bmj.com/content/371/bmj.m4924/rr-6
- https://www.bmj.com/content/371/bmj.m4924/rr-8

40. Proving and Using the Mind in COVID

Many COVID deaths may have been preventable with relatively little effort — many more to come. Meanwhile, we DO have the means for proper research and management.

August 27, 2021

	Daily	Total
Cases worldwide	**712.601**	**216.168.904**
Deaths worldwide	**10.015**	**4.498.140**

The sentiment in large parts of the West

The sentiment is lately one of victory, with the vaccinatory cavalry at our side. It seems like a question of time for the enemy to be defeated. Well, to be more precise, the sentiment is shifting, migrating to "We'll have to live with this." People have become used to COVID.

There is less panic around. But there is more aggression — for instance, between those wanting everybody to wear masks and those resenting masked dictatorship, between those wanting their life and those wanting to live.

Worldwide, there is nothing to celebrate.

Looking at curves from https://www.worldometers.info/:

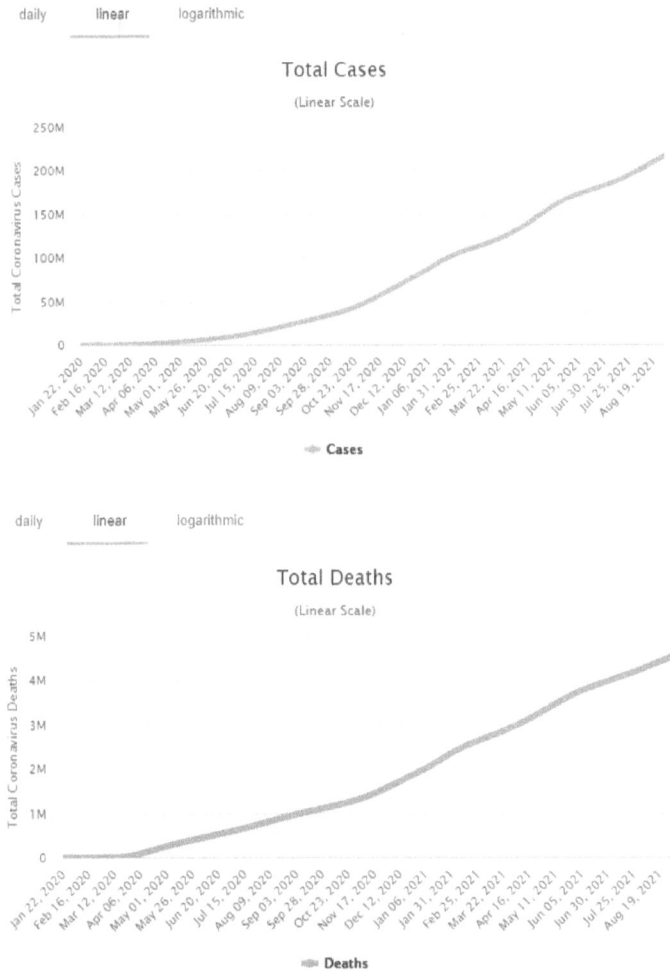

Or take a country like Vietnam:

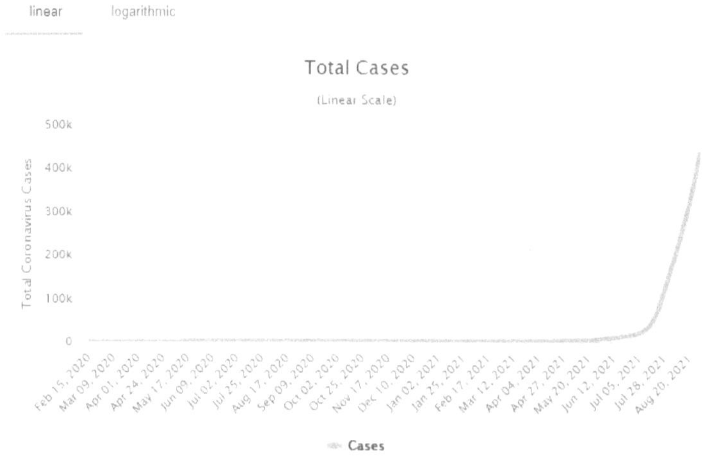

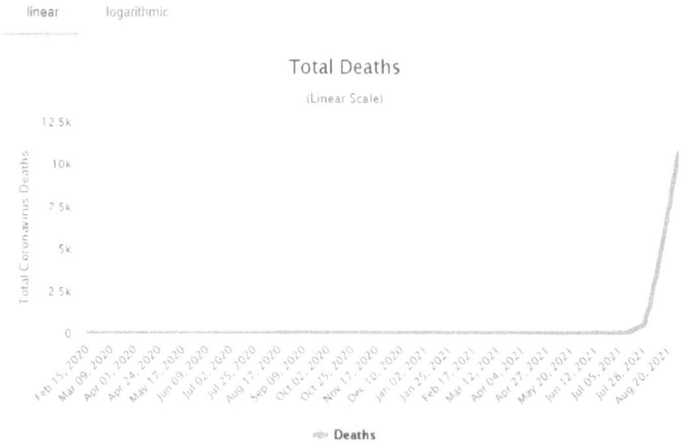

linear   logarithmic

Total Cases

(Linear Scale)

Total Coronavirus Cases

- Cases

linear   logarithmic

Total Deaths

(Linear Scale)

Total Coronavirus Deaths

- Deaths

On top of this, there is the problem of hunger worldwide, with a large uptick due to COVID. According to the World Food Program (WPF), at present, "About **1 billion people** do not have sufficient food consumption in low and lower-middle income countries." From these, 155 million experience acute hunger requiring urgent food, nutrition, and livelihoods assistance. [https://hungermap.wfp.org/?_ga=2.41057058.1433576357.1630347282-559588549.1630347282]

Vaccinatorily

The developers of the vaccines seemed utterly amazed about the efficacy of their products in the initial studies. At the start, they thought about a level of protection at 50%, not 95% (meanwhile, apparently down to 75-85% for the best vaccines).

The high percentages are not astonishing from the hypothesis that this is a 'stress virus.' [see: "Minding COVID: a Different Story"] In the nocebo effect from the start, one can see the human mind in action. In this case, the same action can now be seen in the vaccinations as a diminishing of the nocebo — in a way, the 'placebo of vaccination.' Put this on top of the reasonable 50%, and you may get 90% or more. [see: "What if COVID Vaccinations are 80% Placebo?"]

Meanwhile, there are ways to prove the influence of the mind on COVID progression, individually and in society. There are also ways to come into action based on this proof. The following enumerations are by far not exhaustive.

Three veins of proof

- studies using stress questionnaires and salivary cortisol, for instance, when people enter the hospital (or even before)
- studies using the AURELIS app
- STAT [see: "Why We Need Serial Treatment Assumption Testing"] The 'treatment' in the case of vaccination can be replaced by 'vaccine effectiveness.' This can readily be rolled out even in an extensive study. Of course, no specific company will earn from this — only the whole world, but that doesn't seem to be enough.

How to use the mind in COVID:

- avoiding hyper-anxiety and panic
- avoiding the nocebo of hammering on non-vaccinated state
- using the AURELIS app preventively
- using the AURELIS app at the time of symptom onset or later
- the 'usual protection' (face masks...) also has placebo effects: How to heighten these?

About the disease, some data, and consequences

Three phases in COVID pathophysiology are distinguished:

- early infection: day 0-9
- pulmonary phase: day 9-14
- hyperinflammatory phase: day 14-28…

The symptom onset lies at around day 5.

About the infectious period:

- most infectious: day 4-9
- still pretty infectious: day 9-14

Two consequences of these data

- The infectious period lasts until the start of the hyperinflammatory phase. The peak viral load occurs on average at symptom onset and then steadily declines. As a consequence, the virus doesn't care about the immune-inflammatory over-reaction of its host. Therefore, it doesn't need to attenuate. The virus may become more dangerous to us over time. The delta-variant is an example.
- The symptom onset lies some four days before the pulmonary phase (in 20% of patients), ten days before the hyperinflammatory phase (in 6% of patients). As a consequence, people may get into the COVID-whirlpool, which is most lethal, turbo-charged by nocebo.

Breakthrough cases?

For example, in Connecticut, a US state of 3.6 million people, more than 7,000 COVID breakthrough cases have been reported and 53 deaths until now, by far being driven by the over 75 population. [https://www.nbcconnecticut.com/news/coronavirus/public-health-officials-report-more-than-7000-breakthrough-covid-cases-in-connecticut/2570701/]

That is, relatively seen, not dramatic. However, this is not the corona season.

Transplant this to countries with deficient healthcare, quickly spreading strains, and lower vaccination grades and frequencies, and there's a recipe for more disasters. We just don't know where and when.

Parts of a recent email by me to several people

"As to COVID, with certainty, the mind plays a substantial role. We don't know to what degree. No sound science has been conducted into this anywhere. I've tried to awaken people to this worldwide. Meanwhile, I've learned much about how mind→body is relevant in this domain and why people don't see it (mind-body unity; conceptual-subconceptual; the 'social nocebo' of the global scale).

"About vaccinations: They work (and I've written about how to deeply motivate people to get vaccinated), but we don't know their placebo effect, thus also little about how and when this may tumble down massively. How dangerous this is!!! Variants may be used as an 'excuse' while also being what might suck out confidence — therefore, the placebo itself. The initial vaccination studies were pretty flawed as I, together with some colleagues, have immediately brought forward through some rapid responses in BMJ. I also showed the flawed science about remdesivir half a year before the WHO (submitted to NEJM, not accepted). We showed in this that psychological factors were the probable explanation. Also, we published a rapid response in BMJ about the possible stress-factor in the British variant story, recently scientifically corroborated.

"We are now at 16% vaccination worldwide, an already waning vaccination effectiveness, and daily +/- 10.000 reported deaths (more in reality). What I fear most are multiple vaccine-resistant corona strains being highly transmissible and increasingly adapted to younger ages. Anyway, we cannot be confident that, worldwide, the worst isn't yet to come. My regularly updated book Minding Corona is at 340 pages, the product of +/- a year of 'normal full-time,' unpaid. I also developed a free app, available in app stores, to help people with symptomatic stress and that can be used in research. I did my due.

"Nevertheless, COVID is a relatively small part of what's at stake. Many more healthcare domains lie waiting, not to forget the progress of A.I. itself. We are at a crossroads towards a future of Compassionate A.I. ... or not. See my book."

Silence.

My worst-case scenario a year ago was that some million people would die from COVID. We're already way beyond. Moreover, the worst doesn't come through direct COVID mortality but indirectly through hunger, poverty, and desperation-fueled war situations.

Is this pandemic in reality (that is, not in an academic hide-out) going to take more lives than the one of a century ago?

Will psychological factors eventually show to have had a large causal influence in this?

41. No Psyche in COVID? — Or no COVID Without Psyche?

Sad song

November 5, 2021

	Daily	Total
Cases worldwide	484.847	248.798.420
Deaths worldwide	7.830	5.036.760

Problem

To me, each relatively easily preventable death is shameful.

Since March of 2020, I have been trying to convince medical colleagues and scientists worldwide that the psyche plays a substantial role in COVID progression — in vain.

What would be expected back then is that in due time, epidemiological studies would show relevant correlations. Flash forward to now. Extensive studies on correlations have become feasible. And we see... relevant correlations. More and better studies in the future may reveal more.

540.667

This piece is based on an article of high scientific standard, documenting research from March 2020 to March 2021 over the 'first year of COVID' — pre-vaccination time. [*]

This study examined data from about half a million hospitalized patients from 800 US hospitals, 18 years or older, with COVID-19, based on discharge electronic datasets and using ICD-codes. These don't capture, for instance, 'some feelings of anxiety' but only strong disorders that are recorded as such. In this study, severe COVID was diagnosed when a patient ended up in the intensive care unit, on mechanical ventilation, or died.

Note that these are observational data, in which causality is especially challenging to discern.

These are the results in frequencies of comorbidities from the article:

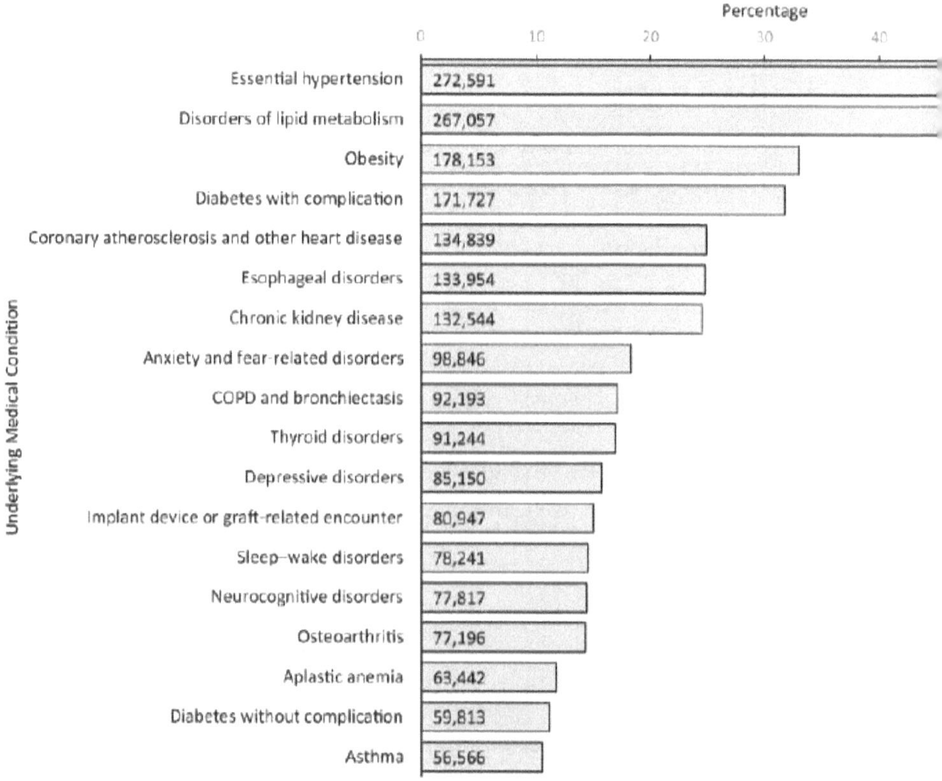

Underlying Medical Condition	Frequency
Essential hypertension	272,591
Disorders of lipid metabolism	267,057
Obesity	178,153
Diabetes with complication	171,727
Coronary atherosclerosis and other heart disease	134,839
Esophageal disorders	133,954
Chronic kidney disease	132,544
Anxiety and fear-related disorders	98,846
COPD and bronchiectasis	92,193
Thyroid disorders	91,244
Depressive disorders	85,150
Implant device or graft-related encounter	80,947
Sleep–wake disorders	78,241
Neurocognitive disorders	77,817
Osteoarthritis	77,196
Aplastic anemia	63,442
Diabetes without complication	59,813
Asthma	56,566

As to the impact on mortality per condition, we see as the top three in the same study:

- obesity: surplus mortality of 30%
- anxiety and fear-related disorders: 28%
- diabetes with complications: 26%

Noteworthy is that depression and several other frequently associated conditions (such as essential hypertension, lipid metabolism disorders, and asthma) somewhat *diminished* the mortality rate. This might be caused by the disorder and/or the therapy, or some bias such as why people are being diagnosed as 'severely ill.' The human body/mind is a highly complex entity. So are diagnosticians.

Anxiety

Strikingly, anxiety shows a substantial correlation with severe COVID illness and death.

Does this mean that some politicians and (social and other) media who did their best to scare people to death in order to make them comply, or just to sell or be in the spotlight, succeeded too literally? This issue should not be easily rejected.

Of course, people may be anxious because of being in the hospital with COVID getting worse. It may also be reciprocal, as in a whirlpool. Also, anxiety being diagnosed before COVID-19 was not independently associated with death or mechanical ventilation during COVID-hospitalization. On the other hand, this does not include much of the direct nocebo effect of being ill with 'the disease.'

As you can see, science is challenging, always. As an intellectual game, it's super. To know the truth, it's the best we've got on the condition that the game is played adequately and with fervor.

What we should do now is take mental profiles/questionnaires and stress parameters such as salivary cortisol of people entering the hospital. This is a pretty blunt instrument but better than nothing for sure. A small Iranian study from March 2020 showed positive results in this. [**] Unfortunately, there has not been any replication of this study as far as I know.

Further remarks

There is more in the data for whoever has some insight in psycho-somatics. If you want a deep dive, you might read my book: [see: "Your Mind As Cure"].

There are immense gaps in our knowledge about causality in several conditions listed above. For instance, there's a reason why essential hypertension is called 'essential.' Meanwhile, there are many severe indications that the mind perspective plays a prominent role in many of them. [see: "Mind the Gap"]

The future of the past

We head towards a future in which this will be apparent, as two centuries ago, we were heading towards a future without leeches and venipunctures.

But surely, now, we have science to guide us, you say? Think again. Indeed, we have proper science oriented towards pharmacology, but not (yet) towards psychotherapy or psycho-somatics. We just haven't, at least not experimentally. As such, we're in the Middle Ages. We can think our way forward, but there is as yet an unfathomable lack of motivation to do so in healthcare. [see: "Are Physicians Interested in Healthcare?"]

10.000.000

Crudely based on US data, it appears that double the numbers of deaths are those of people with 'long-haul COVID.'

That's huge. Many of these may have symptoms for the rest of their lives. Mental problems are substantial in this. And mental causes?

155.000.000

Is   this   number   too   big   to   care?

Worldwide, at present, 155 million people are 'pushed to extreme levels of hunger,' substantially COVID-related (intertwined with conflicts and climate change). [OXFAM]

While we are waging war against the viral enemy, this can be seen as collateral damage. There is no war without it. Starting a war always carries the decision to take such damage for granted. This case is not different. It comes on top of those who directly succumb to COVID. Almost certainly, collateral fatalities are a manifold of the direct deaths.

That's one more reason to not see it as a war but as a jointly Compassionate effort. [see: "The Virus is Not the Enemy"] That makes it all much more human and efficient.

X.000.000.000.000

Several trillion EURO are spent to keep economies afloat after the COVID disaster.

To psychogenic COVID research goes practically nothing.

To feeding the hungry goes way too little.

We have the means for progress.

I mean, some are right under your fingertips, right here. It's ready for scientific studies and to be used in COVID. It's ready for experimentally proving and acting upon what can be done in many healthcare domains. It only needs a diminishment of active denial. [see: "The Basic Denial"]

Is this the complete solution? Surely not.

Is this to be ignored as a decent part of the solution? Surely not.

Should it always at least have been 50/50 in COVID? I think so. What I am sure of is the necessity of sound science in this regard.

One way or another, there is insanity in this.

This insanity doesn't disappear by closing one's eyes or taking refuge in a box.

Please think out of the box.

Seriously.

—

Reference

[*] Kompaniyets L, Pennington AF, Goodman AB, Rosenblum HG, Belay B, Ko JY, Chevinsky JR, Schieber LZ, Summers AD, Lavery AM, Preston LE, Danielson ML, Cui Z, Namulanda G, Yusuf H, Mac Kenzie WR, Wong KK, Baggs J, Boehmer TK, Gundlapalli AV. Underlying Medical Conditions and Severe Illness Among 540,667 Adults Hospitalized With COVID-19, March 2020-March 2021. Prev Chronic Dis. 2021 Jul 1;18:E66. doi: 10.5888/pcd18.210123. PMID: 34197283; PMCID: PMC8269743. You also find the article directly at: https://www.cdc.gov/pcd/issues/2021/21_0123.htm

[**] Ramezani M, Simani L, Karimialavijeh E, Rezaei O, Hajiesmaeili M, Pakdaman H. The Role of Anxiety and Cortisol in Outcomes of Patients With Covid-19. Basic Clin Neurosci. 2020 Mar-Apr;11(2):179-184. doi: 10.32598/bcn.11.covid19.1168.2. Epub 2020 Apr 13. PMID: 32855777; PMCID: PMC7368100.

42. Not Yet Out of the Woods!

The SARS-CoV-2 virus keeps changing, finding new ways for viral success. We're relatively lucky with Omicron. What with the next variant(s)?

January 28, 2022

	Daily	**Total**
Cases worldwide	**3.479.527**	**370.273.350**
Deaths worldwide	**10.595**	**5.667.742**

Curves and numbers

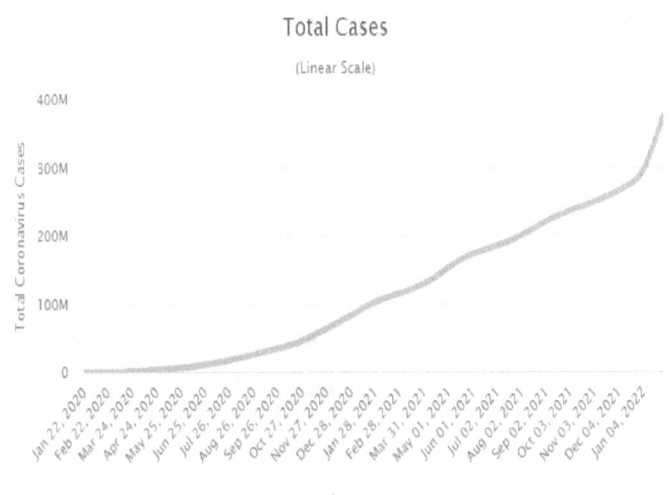

Total Cases

(Linear Scale)

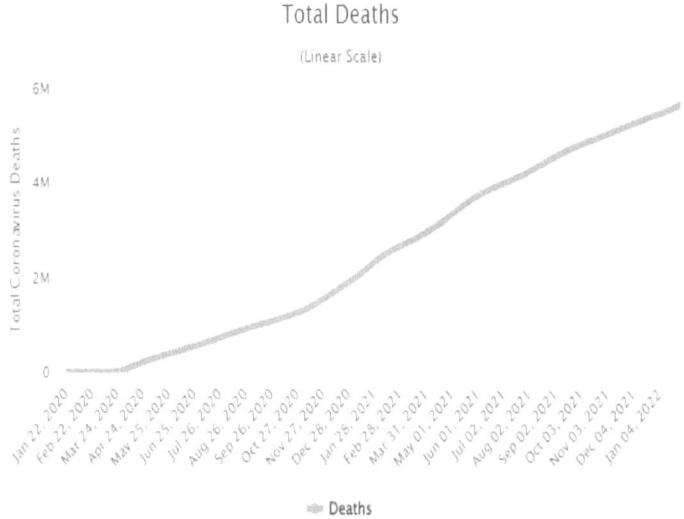

The present week-average mortality lies at 8.732 per day globally. This is higher than the mortality peak of the first wave in 2020, being 7.113. Despite promises (vaccines, drugs), the balance is far worse than average expectations over the whole course. One even gets used to temporary optimism.

I remember a 'lonely poem'.

So, who is winning?

Presently, the virus. Humanity too, since there are so many of us. There are still more people being born than dying.

This is sarcastic indeed. Also sarcastic is the attitude of many who don't seem to care about how many deaths as long as they are personally safe. Each day again, I don't get it.

The genetic landscape of viral fitness

This metaphor – for a map of possible genetic combinations – is not mine. I got it from hearsay, which got it from hearsay. The combinations are purely the result of trial and error. Almost all combinations are errors (meaning reduced fitness), but since there are so many, the chance to hit the jackpot (high level of fitness) is always present.

This is an argument for following safety measures. The argument is not knowing the landscape or the ways at viral disposal to explore it. Within this landscape, there are more or less dangerous regions for us. Some regions are more or less beneficial to the virus. Both kinds of regions are more or less independent from each other.

The danger

The virus moves within this landscape in only slightly predictable ways. For instance, the Omicron variant lies far from the Delta variant within the landscape. This leap was unexpected. Thus, the next one can be equally unexpected, especially since we haven't known this virus long enough to take anything about it for granted.

Meanwhile, the landscape itself keeps changing, rapidly adapting to changes in the landscape. New circumstances are, for instance, the degrees and levels of vaccinations and the immune status of many humans through prior infections. Given the speed of viral change, we can expect it to find new adaptation strategies.

For instance, Omicron found in the human upper airways a relatively little charted part of the landscape with some clear advantages. It very rapidly occupied this part, changing the landscape. The next variant needs a different part, and there are many. Meanwhile, Omicron has shown – again – that SARS-CoV-2 can be a speedy explorer.

The more virus around, the better it can adapt.

Having the virus in all parts of the world and with many people continually moving around globally is very dangerous. Any new viral success gets quickly dispersed, changing the landscape, which invites new viral explorers to discover ever new parts.

And there are many parts in the potential landscape since it is an immense landscape. In principle, viral exploration can go on for a very long time.

Presently, we have the Omicron variant rampaging through Eastern Europe and Russia, as well as South America. The peak in the death toll in those regions is projected within the near future: weeks, maybe months.

As always, the real danger lies in new shifts and drifts — new variants and existing variants adapting to changing circumstances. For instance, more virus leads to quicker vaccine resistance — another argument for following safety measures.

Doesn't the virus take care of us?

Since we are its feeding ground, one would expect the virus to take care not to kill us — no humans, no human coronavirus anymore. Individually seen, if there is no base camp, there can be no jumping over from one to the other.

As said, this virus takes care of the latter by betting on speed: replicating quickly and quickly jumping around. With Omicron, this came together with being less morbid and fatal. We found our ally in that part of the landscape. It may have been sheer luck. The next jump may be an unluckier one.

Doesn't anything else take care of us?

So, if it's that dangerous, one could ask why humans still exist. Why didn't micro-organisms finish us off in the past? Is that not proof of some mechanism (or 'grace') that guards us?

It seems there is this implicit optimism, and I don't want to break it — just trying to stay objective. In the past – a couple of millennia – in Europe, Asia, and North America, huge epidemics have killed almost entire populations. It was not inconceivable for them to be entirely wiped out.

Also, killer viruses may have seen daylight earlier in history, killing all infected. The villages where this happened ceased to exist. At present, the whole world has become one village.

Science might save us. Then again, it might not.

SARS-CoV-2 is an especially rapidly adapting kind of virus.

The Influenza virus, for instance, usually shows 1 or 2 genetic mutations per year in its key protein. The Omicron corona variant has 30 genetic mutations in its key protein in one go.

Also, there is a short interval between infection and infectiousness of only 1.5-3 days. This virus chooses speed over robustness. It can quickly infect many people, which gives it ample room for exploration. After a few days, what happens to the infected person is of little to no concern for the virus. Temporary paralysis of the immune system followed by an overreaction is no problem (for the virus). Viral dreams are about overstressed immune system showing this characteristic.

Why are there waves of infections (past, present, future)?

Influenza comes year after year, predictably sailing a seasonal course. Other viruses (Corona and others) also show such predictability showing up. Where this seasonality comes from is, strangely enough, not well understood. Temperature and humidity play some part. The most significant role may be played by humans, in behavior and more mental aspects.

This includes what people do in private, exhausted of being disciplined, not being given good examples by responsible figures.

Little is known about why exactly many viral presences wax and wane in human populations. Also in this case, although it may be obvious once we see it, there remains much to be learned.

Why the mind is more important than ever.

Many people's faith in materialistic science is not exaggerated, but not always of the correct kind, being rather a faith than science.

Vaccinations seemed like an open door to post-COVID. Until now, it hasn't turned out this way. The situation may have been far worse without vaccinations. Equally obvious is that vaccinations change the viral fitness landscape, and the virus adapts to this changing landscape, searching for new territories. The more changes, the more searching. Eventually, the landscape will be a highly vaccination-driven one.

Present-day vaccinations do not lead to the egg of Columbus. Meanwhile, we still don't know their long-term effects.

New promising drugs are appearing on the market. Good! But giving new antiviral drugs to many people may prove problematic, as in the case of AIDS.

I keep saying that we should take every measure at our disposal, including ourselves.

Also if Omicron shows to be the last main variant and we proceed with small variants upon this one, we may return more readily towards normality – and keep it there – when using our mind.

Science might save us. We need more proper science about us.

43. The Warning of the Virus About Us

Several warnings, eventually. The main one, in my view, is about inner dissociation. We need to get evolving beyond this.
March 1, 2022

	Daily	Total
Cases worldwide	1.633.628	442.061.061
Deaths worldwide	7.777	6.001.323

Read six million deaths until now. It's weird to find it a 'number,' as was, for instance, '40.000' once upon a time. What is in this number? Are there people?

This text is (intended to be) the last chapter of *Minding Corona*. Unfortunately, the main lesson has not been learned; the main warning stays unheeded.

Meanwhile, the virus has not gone at a global scale

although its toll is diminishing in the official reporting. Let's hope this evolution continues, but that is far from certain. Also, COVID may still be raging on in developing countries, hardly officially, as we have not had realistic reporting of them the whole time through. Epidemiologists mention the possibility that the exact numbers of direct COVID-deaths in those countries may be multiple times more.

Then, there are the indirect casualties, the morbidity, and mortality from famine, for instance.

We might be – or better said, are – heading towards new surges.

These may be surges of Corona or, of course, Influenza or another family of viruses. There are lots of eager candidates. COVID has been surprising mainly because many virologists expected other things to happen.

Therefore, the first part of the warning is about whether the mind plays a substantial causal role in any viral infection, or perhaps mainly in any epidemic due to social nocebo effects pushing people into a negative spiral. In this case, we should be doing much research about ourselves in this regard.

"Where is the Mind in COVID-19 Causality?"

I finally succeeded in having a perspective about it – with this title – published in a high-level medical journal (*Brain, Behavior, and Immunity*). This is (and is about) the first time, two years into the COVID disaster, that scientific attention goes to the causal influence of the mind in COVID progression, notwithstanding much indirect evidence.

You find the full article (pdf) from the list of my scientific articles at https://aurelis.org/science-articles.

The promise

The above article is also about the why — mainly focused upon daring. The human being needs to get over the anxiety caused by its predicament. We die. We are not free in the sense that many would like to be. Looking at it more profoundly, this is the promise of the New World. Underlying, it was the promise of the Americas, the land of the free and the brave. From further back in time, it has also been the promise of the New Jerusalem, where people will be eternally happy, free, and unafraid.

This promise will not be attained if people are afraid as if for 'the devil inside' — what may be called 'Eigenangst.' There seems to be a lot of this — and growing. At present, I have no idea where this might end.

COVID is just part of the human story

The question remains: Are 'we' ready for the inner-Copernican revolution that takes the ego out of the center of the universe? Or are 'we' still too afraid of the consequences?

The COVID virus is a stress virus (with its preferred niche of stressed-out organisms). The warning it brings to us is therefore also stress-related. The feeling of stress overlaps with or is the same as inner general anxiety, which is also pretty much the same as the feeling of inner dissociation.

The rest of the path

With so many people on our planet, this has immense consequences in either way towards increasingly more dissociation or Compassion.

Will the following warning be war?

We'll see which journey gets chosen.

Appendices

The COVID-Whirlpool Drawing

(This page is also here in pdf.)

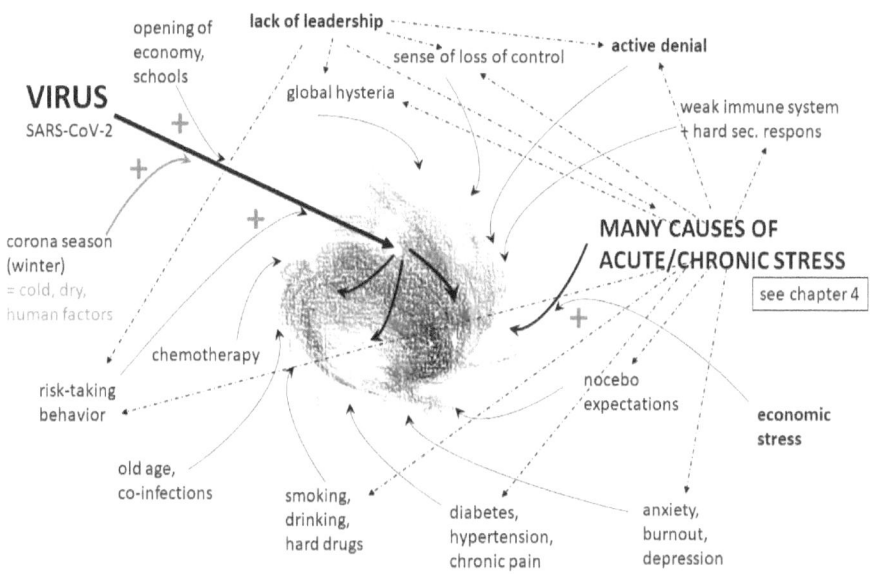

Many elements mutually enforce each other within a self-enhancing whirlpool that individuals and groups are sucked into. The 'energy' within the whole is exponentially much larger than the sum of the distinct elements. Thus, the structure may astonishingly quickly appear, disappear, and reappear. The mind plays a direct role in the whirlpool, as well as in several other factors.

Consequences

- Many health problems (including deaths) and economic mayhem in Europe/US were and are preventable through properly taking the mind into account. Instead, with eyes wide shut, we have collectively fallen into a whirlpool.

- The risk of a second wave in Europe/US is very high, even more so in case of a persistent lack of proper insight into important mind-body influences. Will we fall into this whirlpool again?

- The second wave will probably be larger. We can prevent this by taking appropriate action.

- Disasters in the rest of the world can also be substantially alleviated through the same.

- A more profound lesson about who we are can be learned this way to alleviate and even prevent other disasters in the present and the future.

A primer on nonconscious, subconceptual processing

For more, I refer to the first part of my *Compassionate A.I.*-book and *Your Mind as Cure – Autosuggestion for everyone*. Here's a distillation of some ideas to understand why this issue matters in the whirlpool.

Since we are not computers, we do not have concepts that resemble building blocks in our heads. Instead, we have many neurons and synapses. Each thought, feeling, or motivation comes down to many of these becoming active together, forming a pattern of activity, a distributed set of elements (each being less than a concept, or 'subconceptual'). Patterns may or may not enter consciousness,

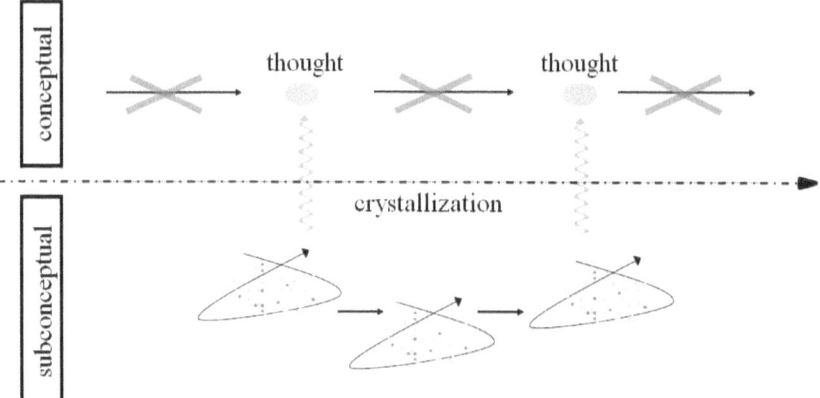

'crystallizing' into concepts. Before they do so, they already influence each other. Any conglomerate of influences is what we perceive as 'meaningful,' or even, depending on circumstances, 'deeply meaningful.' This way, one cannot consciously decide what is personally meaningful, but one can work on it. Doing so in a self-respecting way is what I call autosuggestion.

Beneath the horizontal dashed timeline in this image, you see what happens in the brain/mind, influencing the body because it is the body. Above the line, abstracting away what's beneath, you see what it looks like in conscious awareness. Note that without the lower part, there is no conscious awareness at all, nor a progression from thought to thought. Thus, also, whatever enters the whirlpool does so from below the line.

But this is invisible. It is our basic cognitive illusion to consciously think it's not even there. This illusion makes people vulnerable. We think that we have a control over ourselves that we don't have. On the other hand, there is a possible control that we can cherish and cultivate, but we don't properly do so. In specific circumstances, we are thus prone to inadvertently getting caught in a giant whirlpool, collectively influencing each other deep-to-deep. This way, things may get out of control astonishingly quickly and with most dire consequences.

Not taking into account what's below the line, much effort to manage human affairs is counter-productive. One can see this in many fields of human endeavor. What is perceived as the solution becomes part of the problem. As in this image, one thinks to 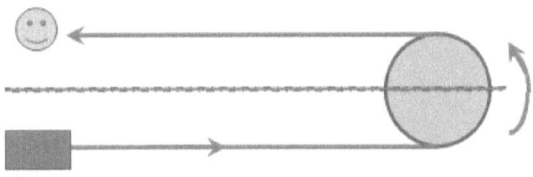 draw the desired result nearer, but the reverse happens. For instance, anticipated motivation becomes demotivation. Fighting stress becomes stressful. Putting more energy into such 'solution' enhances the problem. With some bad luck, this energy additionally fuels the very whirlpool. To alleviate this, or even reverse it, we need to firstly get beyond our basic cognitive illusion individually, collectively, and eventually worldwide. Secondly, we need to treat ourselves and others in Compassionate ways.

Dear reader, if many people cannot be convinced of this, and thus of a *largely preventable* disaster, I give up. In that case, the future even looks bleak for humanity in a few decades.

Lonely Poem

Just let me have a bleeding heart

For those who die alone

In times of corona.

I would like to be with each of them

To die with each of them

So they are not alone.

**

For what is and should not be

Is not one's pain

Is not one's dying

But one's abandonment

To die alone.

**

So let me be with you.

I am your family and friends

Your wife who died a while ago

Your dog, your memories

Your days at the beach when all was well

So you are not alone.

**

As always in suffering

I wonder Where is God?

Did He forget in a blink of His eye

This little planet

Somewhere in His universe?

Or may He be with you

And also die with you

So you are not alone.

*****

One shouldn't analyze a poem. Also, it should not need to be analyzed. A good poem speaks for itself. What it says cannot be put in prose. Otherwise, it would be better to, indeed, put it in prose.

So, these are just some thoughts of mine

The poem was written on March 29, 2020, at a worldwide corona death toll of +/- 40.000.

> [Rereading the poem and this text at a time with a corona death toll of +/- 440.000, the feeling is weird.]

Looking at statistics, people – including me – tend to think of numbers. After a while, a dead person is a dead person. Stars keep on shining. The earth will make its circles around the sun for a while longer. There will be many more deaths.

But this comes different to me. Maybe also to you.

This is about many people presently dying in loneliness. It has probably never happened before on such a scale.

Who can get over it? Who wants to get over it? Is it right to even want to get over it?

Each person can only talk for himself. I can imagine dying in loneliness but will only know it at the end. Still, I want to make a difference between 'alone' and 'lonely.' That might bring some comfort.

One can die alone and yet not be lonely.

The former is physical. The latter is meaningful. Although in the human case, both are intertwined, one can focus a while on the difference in exceptional circumstances. The present may be one. There is no choice in many cases.

Being lonely is being devoid of deepest contact. Being in physical contact is not *necessary* for deepest contact. It is a symbolic happening. It is vertical. In principle, the vertical can exist even without the horizontal. I hope you are following me.

The horizontal can also exist without the vertical. One can be surrounded by people and be lonely.

One can be alone and not be lonely if one feels connected-by-soul (or anything else you want to call it). This being connected-by-soul can be intense. Every human being may have felt this at least once.

This extraordinary time may be an occasion to remember this.

In a way, it lifts the subject of the poem.

There is, of course, no magic involved. One can be perfectly rational and yet remember this.

It happens to be Easter at the time of writing.

Catholics remember Jesus' dying on the cross, in loneliness. Even His last words contain the experience. It's a beautiful poetic story. It is universal. It is very human.

A Tale of Two Letters About Remdesivir

Intrigued by the antiviral drug, remdesivir, I delved into scientific studies about it. The result is a duo of 'Letters to the Editor' to the new England Journal of Medicine (top journal of medical science), in May and June. Not even hoping they would accept, indeed, they didn't. The stakes are too high. The direction too non-mainstream. This way, I can publish it anywhere else. So, after the poetry, I can offer you some science. Note that my credentials are high. I'm not just your average author and I'm perfectly willing to defend my stance in any serious way.

NOTE: According to a preprint on medRxiv, 15 October 2020, of an article by the WHO Solidarity Trial Consortium, remdesivir *"appeared to have little or no effect on hospitalized COVID-19, as indicated by overall mortality, initiation of ventilation and duration of hospital stay. The mortality findings contain most of the randomized evidence on Remdesivir"*

[https://www.medrxiv.org/content/10.1101/2020.10.15.20209817v1]
My intention, five months ago, was not to debunk Remdesivir, but to show the open – yet seemingly invisible – place for the influence of the mind in this research. In order not to see this, one needs to actively look in the other direction. That's worse than blindness.

Here are the two letters:

Remdesivir or 'We,' Which Cure Will it Be?

(submitted May 18, 2020)

Generally, the human mind has no place in causal thinking about COVID-19 progression in the lay press, nor in science. This may be a huge mistake. The exclusive focus lies on material cause and therapies. Even in the latter, the mind may be invisibly intermingled. Making it visible leads to better treatment.

For instance, the Grein study[1], concerning the effect of the broad-spectrum antiviral drug remdesivir on COVID-19, lacks placebo-based randomization. More rigorous studies are being conducted of which fewer than a quarter are double-blind. The most powered and well-conducted research is the ongoing NIAID study, using an inactive placebo (no active ingredients). Preliminary results focus on benefits (mainly, time of recovery) outweighing harms of remdesivir without further concern for the placebo group. In view of the dire need, a second question is more critical than ever: Can the placebo group show us the influence of mind in COVID-19 progression?

Psychoneuroimmunology shows mind-body influences in many health-related domains.[2] There is clear and bidirectional influence of mind on viral diseases.[3] In 2012, we argued a general scheme for understanding mind-related influences of *true* placebo apart from study biases.[4] The second question is as crucial as anything.

How double-blind is a study? Asking patients bluntly to which group they belong, they don't know. Asking them to guess, adverse effects may make them guess correctly. Double-blindness strives also to eliminate unconscious influences from testing result. Therefore, we need to look also at unconscious blindness, especially in suggestible circumstances and immense stress. One needs not to look further. In the [Grein et al., 2020] study, adverse effects (increased hepatic enzymes, diarrhea, rashes, renal impairment, hypotension) were reported in 60% of patients. This makes double-blindness doubtful, heightening blindness to the relative effect of mind in *both* study groups. We deserve better especially now.

A vaccine may still take a long time to be developed. No therapies for COVID-19 have been adequate to date. Remdesivir may have some effect, but little and at a considerable cost (adverse reactions). A *true* placebo effect would show that mind-related factors play a significant role, as is theoretically probable. Knowing about mind-COVID influence may inspire health-promoting communications. Tools can be made available at a grand scale for individual help. A.I. can be integrated towards enhancing these tools and towards input of real-world scientific data. Lives can be saved. Making social contacts safer this way may significantly impact the economy and flatten disasters also in countries like India and Brazil.

References

1. Grein J, Ohmagari N, Shin D, et al. Compassionate Use of Remdesivir for Patients with Severe COVID-19 [published online ahead of print, 2020 Apr 10]. *N Engl J Med*. 2020;NEJMoa2007016.

2. Segerstrom SC, Miller GE. Psychological stress and the human immune system: a meta-analytic study of 30 years of inquiry. *Psychol Bull*. 2004;130(4):601–63.

3. Coughlin SS. Anxiety and Depression: Linkages with Viral Diseases. *Public Health Rev*. 2012;34(2):92.

4. Mommaerts JL, Devroey D. The placebo effect: how the subconscious fits in. *Perspect Biol Med*. 2012;55(1):43-58.

Enter Mind – Exit Remdesivir?

(submitted June 4, 2020)

Letter to the editor in reference to: Beigel JH, Tomashek KM, Dodd LE, et al. Remdesivir for the Treatment of COVID-19 - Preliminary Report [published online ahead of print, 2020 May 22]. *N Engl J Med*. 2020;10.1056/NEJMoa2007764. doi:10.1056/NEJMoa2007764

The prematurely finished remdesivir-trial published by Beigel et al.[1] may prove that mind, not remdesivir, influences COVID-19 progression.

Infusion reactions have been noted shortly after administration[2], influencing patients' treatment assumptions, enhanced through daily kindling, breaking double-blind. With patients knowing when they received some product[1], we refer to hidden-administration trials where effects are grossly dependent on such patient knowledge[3]. Remdesivir heightens transaminases up to 20-fold[2], patients with already high transaminases being excluded[2]. This suggests the correct group allocation to caregivers, breaking double-blind. Moreover, all placebos were passive[2].

The baseline-5 group is arguably most suggestible. Here lies the positive effect of remdesivir-administration in contrast to other groups, most intriguingly baseline-7. Apparently, for remdesivir-administration to work, patients are necessarily fully conscious. This, together with a counter-intuitive effect from day one, may show the effectiveness not of remdesivir, but of the mind.

We hypothesize that the absence of mind in COVID-19 causal thinking cost many more lives than remdesivir could ever save. We urge appropriate research. It would be devastating to see the need for this only in retrospect.

References

(1) Beigel JH, Tomashek KM, Dodd LE, et al. Remdesivir for the Treatment of COVID-19 - Preliminary Report [published online ahead of print, 2020 May 22]. *N Engl J Med.* 2020;10.1056/NEJMoa2007764. doi:10.1056/NEJMoa2007764

(2) Fact Sheet for Healthcare Providers - Emergency Use Authorization (EUA) of Remdesivir (GS-5734TM) [Internet]. U.S. Food and Drug Administration (FDA). 2020. Available from: www.fda.gov/media/137566/download

(3) Benedetti F, Carlino E, Pollo A. Hidden administration of drugs. *Clin Pharmacol Ther*. 2011;90(5):651-661. doi:10.1038/clpt.2011.206

Why and How to Wear a Face Mask

There is a difference between motivation and coercion, even when using scientific arguments. If one wants people — including oneself — to wear and continue wearing face masks, one needs to motivate them. This is: to provide them with the means by which they can motivate themselves. There is no other way. Besides, it's an interesting way.

20 reasons, more or less frivolous

- It's not comfortable, but you don't care.
- You can express your individuality (facemask fashion).
- It draws attention to your eyes.
- It opens jobs and shops.
- You decide it yourself, even if.
- You don't need to know people to care for them.
- You can feel fine in it, after all.
- You forgot to take it off.
- It is cool if you make it so.
- You are loyal to your species.
- You've made wearing it your new habit.
- Somehow, sometimes, you find it erotic.
- You make others less anxious.
- You've learned to be proud of wearing one.
- It unites against the viral enemy.

- Yours is beautiful (mine is black).

- The heavy breathing makes you stronger.

- You can un-wear it under the shower.

- Old people are fabulous.

- That's the way God protects you.

Seriously

Of course, some of the reasons on the list are not frivolous at all. I see in them that some reasons can be frivolous or even incomprehensible to some people while being of deadly earnest to others. We should leave for anybody to know or feel the reasons why.

Also, we should give proper attention to the reasons why not. The cons are not necessarily bad people. As a physician, I can only say that from the standpoint of physical health, the recommendation is to wear them. But even so, health is not the only value; neither is it a strict value. There is no definition of health that can be imposed on all people. Health is what we make of it. It is not simply the absence of disease. In *Your Mind as Cure*, I idiosyncratically define it as the ability to change and to enjoy.

In the case of face masks, this broader take on health may enable pros and cons (and all in-betweens) to at least better understand each other. For the pros: simply juggling with science as if this says everything there is to say, will not motivate those cons who feel that you are hiding behind a strictness to which reality does not accord. The best science, of course, takes into account the whole of reality. We don't need less science. We only need more, and more encompassing. This way, the dialogue can have more rational arguments to which (almost) everybody listens or doesn't immediately run away from. Also, there will be less chance for manipulators to do their sorry thing.

So, please be aware that this viral disease takes many dead and wounded. With wounded, I mean those who suffer from complications that may last a lifetime. What also holds my attention is the risk of viral mutation. The

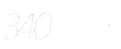

more people infected, the higher are the chances of a mutation into an even deadlier strain. This way, we are all somewhat responsible for all on this planet. I hope this fear will not materialize as it did with the previous comparable pandemic a century ago. One cannot rule it out. The death toll may, from that moment, rise to x 10.

It's a sunny day today. There are no viruses to be spotted. There are children playing in gardens and at beaches. We live on a time bomb that might go off on top of the already present worldwide disaster – not even talking about the whirlpool. It's challenging to combine things. It's difficult to not succumb to paralyzing disgust. We all go our ways.

It is a proven fact that wearing face masks leads to less COVID. From a conceptual viewpoint, it is logical why: fewer viruses in the air, less contagion, less disease. However, it is not proven that this is the complete answer. By wearing a mask, one shows to others that one cares. Really. It heightens the idea of us all caring together and going to make it. With a pair of friendly eyes above the mask, the message is one of Compassion. This is what I call a deep-to-deep communication that may diminish the negative energy of the whirlpool. Every contact in social distancing can be a message of social togetherness. In my view, the influence of this is profound, having a positive impact on the giver's and receiver's immune system. To me, then, it's a beautiful world despite the virus, after all. I speak for myself. I long for such.

Looking at reasons for not wearing a face mask, I see many, some of which are quite ego-bound, others not so much. One may prefer living life in danger above not living life at all. One may hold specific principles higher than health.

We are all in this together, whether we like it or not, with our different values and principles. No-one only decides for himself; every decision involves the wellbeing of others, and vice versa. In this sense, what should be done by all is not to look at oneself as the only worthwhile person on earth, nor one's bubble as the single worthwhile bubble. I know: saying this already holds a personal value. It is my value. I want to take care of myself as well as many others. Moreover, I want to do so regarding total persons, not mere ego-ness. Sometimes, this leads to specific choices.

Still, people may want to run around with naked noses and mouths all the time. One way or another, this leads to a longer-lasting pandemic. Which is worth what? In any case, it is worthwhile to look at your values again and again. What do they mean? Do you find common humanity in them?

In your reasons for not wearing this piece of cloth, can you still find underlying reasons for wearing it? In the 'frivolous' reasons, you may find some examples.

This might make us all better human beings, not by being coerced in any way, but by finding our humanity in what has been and what becomes, so we can all be proud of what is behind our masks. I think this may be the best reason for wearing one and also the best way how to wear it: with pride.

Masked Poetry

For the doctors and nurses
Who give more than ever you can
Please put on your mask.

For the beauty of eyes
That are looking at a beautiful world
From right above a mask,

For your parents and grandparents
Who want to keep getting your love
Keep on that face mask.

For your children and grandchildren,
For a future we all want to
Live in without any mask,

For the caregivers in homes
Who do not deserve the next wave
Keep wearing your face mask.

For those you don't know
Who suffer in a much poorer world
Wearing a quite different mask,

MINDING CORONA

For a friendly new world
For seeing each other more deeply inside
Don't take off your mask.

For a merciful Compassionate God
Whom you may happen to believe in
Asking to wear this mask,

For these misguided viruses even
Who never have wanted to hurt anyone
They too want your mask.

For the people I love
And want to touch again pretty soon
Don't ever forget that mask.

Face Mask Meditation

Wearing a face mask during formal group-meditation may be less comfortable. It may also be more interesting.

Readers may know me as a meditator

I am a very inconsistent one. Sometimes, I go to a group for 'formal meditation' on a cushion. Sometimes, I go to a seven-day meditation. I would like to go more but don't take the time. I write too much.

In COVID times, in a group

Meditation is freedom. All is possible; no coercion. At the same time, meditation is discipline. This comes from inside out. No discipline, no meditation. Maybe some daydreaming or some look-at-me, but no meditation.

Again, no coercion, so, there should not be any coercion to wear a mask. There is also no coercion to stay somewhere in group meditation if some people don't wear a face mask. It's simple: no coercion in any way at all.

At least, of course, that's my idea of the happening.

This makes wearing a face mask very interesting in meditation

We're not talking about you on your lonely cellar or in your garden. We're talking in group. Or, maybe better, just not talking too much anyway. Just the necessary.

Then a face mask is like a thought that comes to disturb you. In meditation, specific attention goes to such thoughts (called bonnos in some tradition). Of course, every meditator knows that such disturbing thoughts are present most of the time. Or are they not?

The face mask may feel like a disturbing thought. You sit and wear one, and it's there, and it's there. And sometimes, it's gone, and then it's there, again. Right. How to meditate with a face mask sticking on your face all the way?

Not the mask disturbs, but the interpretation of the meditator. Without the interpretation, the face mask wouldn't disturb at all. And that makes it very interesting.

Interesting, how?

Because it's you. The face mask is not you. Your interpretation is you. It is who you are. So, being in contact with your interpretation can teach you a lot about you, as a meditator, and a person who, through this, may become a better person.

As a superficial thought, your (interpretation of your) face mask may disturb you. Your attention goes to the disturbance. The meditation doesn't work optimally. So, even more attention goes to the disturbance. You know where I'm getting at.

You can put the face mask beside you. Hm. You can put the disturbing thought beside you. Again, hm. That's not interesting. It's just getting rid of something. You lose a chance, a contact, a communication, a path to your inner strength, a heavenly road to deep meditation.

A disturbing thought comes to you because it's interesting to you. A disturbing interpretation of a face mask hits you in the face because it's interesting to you. What does it tell you? Listen. Keep listening. Keep listening deeply. Then it may bring you to the other side.

This is also the other side of attention: superficial versus deep.

To many people, the concept of deep attention is a difficult one. That is understandable. Well, this is an occasion to learn. Not easy at all! This is what meditation is for in the first place. Not to feel good, but to feel bad in such a deep way that it feels good. Then to feel good in such a deep way that it also feels good like any other good feeling is hardly comparable to this. The bad feeling is not interesting as such. Even the good feeling is not interesting as such. The deep way is interesting.

This way also, you can learn to wear a face mask on other occasions as something that can be interesting in many ways, for instance, out of Friendliness.

We will need to wear it for a very, very long time to come. We can better learn to see this not as a disturbance to get rid of, but an asset.

Minding COVID: a Different Story

May 10, 2020

[This is a general text, not written in the succession of the other chapters. This one is written to give new readers a wide-ranging overview. Thus, there is some overlap in this one versus the other chapters.]

The human mind is missing in the causal story of COVID. Putting it in place makes a Different Story. This is a story about a virus, but even more is it a story about humankind.

Where is the human mind in the causal story of COVID? It is not in the media, nor the scientific literature. It is not in the minds of most people. Of course, there is a lot of talk about mind in consequence: the loneliness, the aggression, the depression, the immediate and post-traumatic stress. This will become even more so after the first shockwave of disease when we get into a prolonged presence of COVID in smaller waves. In the causal story, we don't see it now.

And yet **these are certainties**:

- The immune system plays a significant role in the causal story of COVID-progression in any individual.
- The mind plays a significant role in immune reactions – and other defense mechanisms.

Straightforwardly, the mind should be at the center stage. Then why is it invisible in the causal storytelling? Part of the answer is mundane: precisely because it's invisible as such. One cannot see it because it is the thing with which is being seen. Even when opening the skull, one cannot see the mind. When looking at the world, we actually see only its interaction with our mind. Thus, to be more precise, we are partly looking at mind all the time. Yet we have a hard time seeing things this way. Ironically, this blinds us to our blindness. It blinds us also to our own capabilities.

The invisibility in any kind of media is unfortunate. With a virus wreaking havoc in the present and near-future, we should call all hands on deck. Yet there is an utter silence regarding mind. Why? Besides being visibly invisible, there are **two rather underlying long-time reasons why mind does not enter the causal story:**

1. the wrongful supposition that body and mind are two distinct entities

    So, how would the *ephemeral* mind be able to influence the material body?

    >< Mind and body are two ways of looking at the same thing.

2. the wrongful supposition that mind only exists in conscious awareness.

    So, how would the *conscious* mind be able to influence the body? This seems like a two-dimensions-distance this way.

    >< Every conscious thought, feeling, motivation is the result of non-conscious processing.

Both suppositions, at least in a stark formulation, flourished from the mind of the French philosopher René Descartes (1596-1650). They were signs of coming times. Both ideas have thoroughly influenced Western culture, including modern medicine. Meanwhile, science has shown with utmost certainty that both suppositions are wrong. But **getting beyond them comes at huge costs** to the individual (especially in mere-ego), respectively:

1. This means that together with the death of the body comes the end of mind as we know it. Note that this is not necessarily related to the 'soul.' What we know is that the mind changes with the body and dies with the body.

2. This means that 'conscious free will' is mainly an illusion. A lot of non-conscious meaningful stuff is at the origin of any of our thoughts, feelings, motivations.

Both costs can provoke a lot of anxiety, which contributes to why they are vehemently shunned. On the other side, one can **look at the refutations of the presuppositions from a positive viewpoint.** Again, respectively:

1. The mind can be used to work on better health, including that of the body. There is a lot of therapeutic potential in this. We have only scraped at the surface.

2. There is a lot of potential for inner growth. The mind is much broader than is generally conceived. This growth can be human-potential-oriented, as in art, in-depth communication, coaching. Here still lies a lot to be done.

Because of the – untoward – invisibility and the above suppositions (together with money and status issues), **it is daring for anyone to come forward** with the idea that the mind is deeply involved in the huge catastrophe that is befalling large parts of the world. An additional danger is that people may push all kinds of unscientific ideas about mind in this respect. Coming forward with mind-as-cause will, to many, also link the one who rationally does so with those doing so from nonscientific hypotheses. We can better be prepared and bring science at its best. Only top-notch science – taking into account the total person in a realistic manner – can save us from a swamp of absurdity. This is a shared responsibility.

To see the unity of body and mind, one needs to see that this is not merely related to conscious awareness. For instance, **I cannot choose to blush by conscious decision**. Yet something meaningful happens, and I may blush. The meaning is mind-related. The blushing is visible in my body.

Of course, the impact of **what is meaning-related goes much deeper than the skin.** In an acute meaningful situation, my blood pressure may rise, and my autonomic nervous system shows many complex reactions. Also, my brain reacts in a myriad of ways, sending more blood to this part, abstaining from that part. Neurotransmitters and other brain messenger molecules get into a complex intermingle. My body influences my brain and vice versa.

This is about acute meaningfulness. Anyone may experience the consequences. **In a chronic situation, it is more challenging to see body-mind-unity.** Especially in experimental science, it is much harder to pinpoint. There is the complexity of the ever-changing situation as well as of body and mind, and dynamic meaningfulness. What something meant to me yesterday does not necessarily mean the same tomorrow. What is stressing (or not) also changes with meaningfulness.

Even so, **we doubtlessly know that chronic stress can have a detrimental influence** on the immune system and chronic inflammation. Logically, this paves the way for a worse outcome in case of any acute superposition. The chronic stress has weakened the person. The acute gives a blow that sometimes cannot be handled. A subsequent illness from a viral infection, even death, can be the result.

The mind significantly influences the body in sickness and healing in ways that are relevant in times of COVID. We know scientifically that mental stress can lead to chronic or acute inflammation, even provoking instant death as in the case of the heart disease 'takotsubo' [1]. In dermatology, we clearly see the acute and chronic effects of mental stress on skin diseases [2]. Of course, what we see on the outside happens likewise on the inside. Mental stress influence on lung tissue inflammation has also been described. Ring a bell?

A few quotes from PubMed (top scientific medical journal) articles might be intriguing to you:

- "The studies summarized in this review indicate that there are important linkages between anxiety and depression and viral diseases such as influenza A (H1N1) and other influenza viruses, varicella-zoster virus, herpes simplex virus, human immunodeficiency virus/acquired immune deficiency syndrome, and hepatitis C." [3]

- "The present report meta-analyzes more than 300 empirical articles describing a relationship between psychological stress and parameters of the immune system in human participants. Acute stressors (lasting minutes) were associated with potentially adaptive upregulation of some parameters of natural immunity and downregulation of some functions of specific immunity. Brief naturalistic stressors (such as exams) tended to suppress cellular immunity while preserving humoral immunity. Chronic stressors were associated with suppression of both cellular and humoral measures." [4]

- "Cortisol also showed a continuous association with duration of viral shedding, an indicator of viral replication and continuing infection, such that higher cortisol concentrations predicted more days of shedding." [5]

- "Both aging processes and psychological stress affect the immune system: Each can dysregulate immune function with a potentially substantial impact on physical health. Worse, the effects of stress and age are interactive." [6]

- "Stress-induced immune dysregulation has been shown to be significant enough to result in health consequences, including reducing the immune response to vaccines, slowing wound healing, reactivating latent herpesviruses, such as Epstein-Barr virus (EBV), and enhancing the risk for more severe infectious disease." [7]

- "Importantly, we concluded that nocebo studies outline how individual expectations may lead to physiological changes underpinning the central integration and processing of magnified pain signaling." [8]

- "Stress is an external factor known to be a potent exacerbator of respiratory infections. Most explanations of how stress affects susceptibility to airway infections focus on the immune system. However, evidence is increasing that respiratory pathogens are equally responsive to the hormonal output of stress." [9]

- "Media reports about the adverse effects of supposedly hazardous substances can increase the likelihood of experiencing symptoms following sham exposure and developing an apparent sensitivity to it." [10]

These are just a few examples. Moreover, we have scientifically started to look with special scanners into the brain and deeper mind, as well described, for instance, by David Eagleman [11]. We have scientifically started *seeing* it happen. **Then why – in any causal sense – is the mind, let alone deeper mind, nowhere in the news while the virus is everywhere in the news?**

Of course, even more broadly, non-conscious processing is little in sight. Yet be honest: Where does any of your spontaneous thoughts come from? Not from the sky, not from sheer coincidence. It can only come from your deeper mind. To see this, you just need to stretch your arm. Look at your thumbnail. This is the area that you see in focus in any normal circumstance. Yet typically, it seems like everything is in focus. This is an illusion. Likewise, you may think that you can have everything in your mind in conscious focus. That is also an illusion. Most of it, you principally *never* have in focus. Meanwhile, it is there, and it determines you in many ways, including your immune system. Thus:

> **Concerning COVID-19 (the disease, not the infection): the mind may be considerably important, alongside the virus, in its cause as well as proper management.**

A short sentence, an immense implication.

Science is unmistakable. Mind can and does play a significant role in many cases of viral-disease-progression. Thus, most probably also in the present case. In the future, to deny this may be looked upon as a crime. Taking it into account at present can alleviate a lot of physical suffering and economic hardship. This does not banalize what is happening. On the contrary, we should stop banalizing our mind. To do so, we need to get beyond the above suppositions. That takes courage. The reward – as a worldwide society – is immense.

What probably happens in COVID-progression is that the **immune system responds too late, then over-shoots with a lot of inflammatory reaction.** Many deaths are the result of the latter. Here, things fit together. The virus attacks and lets itself be replicated like crazy in the short term. The person gets very contagious, transmitting the virus before the immune response comes like a thunderbolt. When it comes, it may kill the person, but transmission is completed. The virus has found this – by happenstance, of course – as its niche. This niche is hugely stress-related – not the stress of a simple stress-o-meter score but of deep meaningfulness. Remember the body-mind-unity and the impact of chronic meaningfulness. An additional problem is: We have a body made for acute stress and a mind that provokes chronic stress in circumstances and interpretations, regularly ruminating and projecting all kinds of stressful thoughts. This makes us vulnerable. On the other side, we can use our complex minds in many positive ways.

Now let's go into the **science about 'mind on corona.'** Optimistically, I went for a search on PubMed on 18 March 2020, searching for 'COVID' and 'coronavirus' separately. Note that 'coronavirus' also comprises SARS and MERS, separate from COVID-19. The results were as follows:

Search term	Number of articles found
COVID/coronavirus psychosocial	0
COVID/coronavirus depression	0
COVID/coronavirus social stress	0
COVID/coronavirus psychological	0
COVID/coronavirus psychology	0
COVID/coronavirus mental	0

Also, nothing related that I could think of. The whole domain doesn't look mind-related because no one mentions it. Therefore, no one mentions it.

Yet, other research is more than clear. This includes – crucial to the present case of COVID – unmistakable proof of influence of psychosocial stress on immuno-inflammatory mechanisms as measured in saliva and in the blood.

Scientifically studied mental factors influencing immunology include chronic stress, depression, anxiety, aggression, social deprivation, mourning, a feeling of powerlessness, and uncertainty. Scientific data support all of these influences, clearly, firmly, and robustly. Note that they are all familiar factors in recent times. They are all intensified by lockdown. We have a mental situation that conduces to sharpen the progression of COVID. With more proper distinctions being made in mental factors, the future is bound to show more. Of course, this does not mean that we should lessen social distancing for as long as needed. At least, we need to bring it about with proper motivation.

These insights can help us **see COVID not as a disease singly caused by a virus but a whirlpool of factors** in which the virus 'only' plays an important role. This makes one more sensitive to how and why other factors can better be handled. Our own complexity (mind – immune – inflammation) is also present in the whirlpool. Being singularly focused on the 'virus as enemy' makes us blind to the whirlpool. The virus is inside it, as are panicky thoughts and many meaningful elements. Even the readiness for 'waging war against the virus,' if mingled with aggressive undertones, can be a nasty element in the whirlpool. It is cause and consequence, as is the whirlpool itself. As the only element, the virus would possibly not be very energetic in this whirlpool. But combine it with much harmful mental content, and the whole may grab you, then make you ill and eventually kill. Yet from outside the whirlpool, only the virus is visible to many. That is an illusion. A patient who gets into the whirlpool bears the consequences. Before getting stuck in it, not much may be needed to keep out. When inside, the mind may be used to avoid worse.

This does not demean the worthy actions of caregivers. On the contrary, it highlights their immense importance as human beings on top of medical expertise. Moreover, it may relieve their burden in several ways.

Caregivers and patients may work even more together as 'brothers in arms.' They fight for health and healing, not simply against an invisible demon. Secondly, caregivers too may work on not getting in the whirlpool. They are a population at risk, of course. This way, patient and caregiver share experiences. Thirdly, if people can prevent getting into the whirlpool, this is good for everybody. Fourthly, every patient who recovers is a source of joy for the caregivers too. It all makes their work more rewarding.

Mind over COVID: the Different Story is at first place a different view upon ourselves. For humanity, this transcends the present disaster. We see several crises getting worse over the years and in many domains. We rave about politics, economics, divides of many kinds. In all domains, the prime divide is internal: between who we consciously think we are and who we really are. We may fill this divide like filling with mud (such as the two wrongful suppositions) many cracks in a house while the house itself is falling apart. It takes a storm to show this more clearly, but the storm is not initially causing it. The internal divide makes one look for any externality – the enemy of any kind, the bad guys, the threatening ones, the not-us-and-therefore-them, the storms themselves – as explanations for what we don't see because it's invisible.

Are most people ready for the necessary insight? Probably not, and that is scary. It's also a pity, but there is no time for a most gentle slope toward readiness. Also, part of the problem is the non-readiness itself. Waiting for the solution to tackle the problem, will never solve the problem. So better work on it continuously, including now, even while it may be said that "there is no time to waste in a battle against the virus." That seems to be like going to war without any personal protection because "there is no time to waste." That is just a silly thing to do.

People are not machines. They are in-depth treated too much as such in economics, in medicine, in clinical psychology, in everything human-related. As a result, we are stuck in a pseudo-rationalized world. We have lost nature-within-ourselves. The virus didn't come to show us so. It just found a niche, created by us. This can also attract other mishaps. Is this an inconvenient message? Yes. So, will we need to see in hindsight of COVID that we have again been looking past ourselves on the way towards a next disaster? Humanity should have progressed further. This is a failure and, above all, not to be continued. We need to get to know ourselves. COVID is but a part of the reason why. In our ever more complex world, there will be more and harsher reasons. And indeed, they are already present or in the making. For instance, a pandemic of depression and burnout. Or, for example, a future of Compassion-less A.I. We should not forget how quickly this COVID-wave came out of the blue sky. Let's learn the deeper lesson, not in the sense of "This or that should be done," but an invitation to live this life profoundly. The Different Story may still be a beautiful one. **This is about the human being who gets to know oneself as total person.**

References

[1] Dawson DK. Acute stress-induced (takotsubo) cardiomyopathy. *Heart*. 2018;104(2):96–102.

[2] Marshall C, Taylor R, Bewley A. Psychodermatology in Clinical Practice: Main Principles. Acta Derm Venereol. 2016;96(217):30–34.

[3] Coughlin SS. Anxiety and Depression: Linkages with Viral Diseases. *Public Health Rev*. 2012;34(2):92.

[4] Segerstrom SC, Miller GE. Psychological stress and the human immune system: a meta-analytic study of 30 years of inquiry. *Psychol Bull*. 2004;130(4):601–630.

[5] Janicki-Deverts D, Cohen S, Turner RB, Doyle WJ. Basal salivary cortisol secretion and susceptibility to upper respiratory infection. *Brain Behav Immun*. 2016;53:255–261.

[6] Graham JE, Christian LM, Kiecolt-Glaser JK. Stress, age, and immune function: toward a lifespan approach. *J Behav Med*. 2006;29(4):389–400. doi:10.1007/s10865-006-9057-4.

[7] Godbout JP, Glaser R. Stress-induced immune dysregulation: implications for wound healing, infectious disease and cancer. *J Neuroimmune Pharmacol*. 2006;1(4):421–427.

[8] Blasini M, Corsi N, Klinger R, Colloca L. Nocebo and pain: An overview of the psychoneurobiological mechanisms. *Pain Rep*. 2017;2(2):e585.

[9] Stover CM. Mechanisms of Stress-Mediated Modulation of Upper and Lower Respiratory Tract Infections. *Adv Exp Med Biol*. 2016;874:215–223.

[10] Witthöft M, Rubin GJ. Are media warnings about the adverse health effects of modern life self-fulfilling? An experimental study on idiopathic environmental intolerance attributed to electromagnetic fields (IEI-EMF). *J Psychosom Res*. 2013;74(3):206–212.

[11] Eagleman D. The Brain: The Story of You. Canongate Books Ltd, Edinburgh, GB 2015.

The Future of the COVID Story

August 1, 2020

I started writing MINDING CORONA in March 2020, with 12 points. They're still valid. After five months, of course, we know a bit more about the future. So, I can recapitulate and see what is bound to happen.

The near future is grim. Not wanting to see it doesn't make it less grim. Looking at it straight on helps to find additional solutions that can make a huge difference.

In 12 bullet points, very succinctly:

1. The COVID-virus is here to stay, principally forever.
2. It will hardly attenuate, since it has no reason to, contrary to other viruses.
3. There will be very many long-term health complications.
4. A proper vaccine is bound to be available around mid-2021. Don't expect it to be a miracle cure.
5. Medical treatment will ameliorate over the years. Till then, we have to get used to face masks.
6. In developing countries, the misery will continue much longer and take many more deaths due to COVID and other diseases, hunger, and general lack of resources.
7. We are flying on one wing, namely the conceptual one, looking mainly at the virus as an enemy.

8. The other wing (our mind) is very much a burden at present. Not seeing the COVID-whirlpool, there are dangerous surprises ahead.

9. We can make this other wing into a VERY POSITIVE ASSET right now. [see: "Free App to Relieve COVID"]

10. If we don't, there will be more deaths in the future than in the past.

11. In that case, the economic consequence of what will be is bound to be harsher than that of what has been until now.

12. Artificial Intelligence carries much promise towards further support in using our second wing.

As to mind-body-unity and all the ramifications of implications, it's as if we are still in an era of pre-science. No more than two centuries ago, the regular medicine of that time was still very much into bloodletting, leeches, enemas, scarifications... in a theory of four humours that has since been entirely surpassed. Good! Imagine being a physician back then but with the knowledge of now. Hmm. As to the mind, at present, we still have a very long way to go. COVID might be an occasion to warp us towards a future of better science in this domain. To read more about this, see Your Mind as Cure.

New Strain or Brexit Stress?

Big news on +/- December 18, 2020, two weeks before hard Brexit hangs in the winter air: "If a new virus sounds scary, a new mutating virus sounds scarier still. In Kent in September, scientists now believe, somebody with Covid was the unlucky first person to pass on a variant form of the coronavirus that is maybe as much as 70% more transmissible than the version we have been used to. The exponential recent rise in cases now blamed on that incident and the UK government response have sparked alarm around the world." [https://www.theguardian.com/world/2020/dec/21/new-covid-variant-in-uk-spreading-christmas-fear]

Let's look into three hypotheses for what happened:

- Hypothesis 1: A new and more transmissible strain of the virus is detected in the Southeast of the UK. This strain causes an upsurge in the number of infected people who fortunately don't appear to become more ill through infection.
- Hypothesis 2: Pure chance or coincidence: According to (Australian) Victoria's deputy chief health officer, Prof Allen Cheng, "It was not clear whether the UK variant was truly more infectious. It could appear to be spreading faster for multiple reasons. For example, it could be simply the strain that was involved in a super-spreading event, or spreading in a part of the country where restrictions are less strict or less adhered to. Higher viral loads could reflect detection earlier in the illness." [https://www.theguardian.com/world/2020/dec/21/australian-health-officials-cast-doubt-on-claim-new-uk-covid-strain-more-infectious]
- Hypothesis 3: A mass hysterical reaction in the Southeast of the UK, including London, co-engendered by Brexit mishap, makes people more suggestible, vulnerable to nocebo [see chapter: "Is

Social Nocebo Real?"] and vigilance to the symptoms of the viral disease that presently also has a huge symbolic meaning to many people. A stressed immune system is more vulnerable to COVID, whereby people may become more ill and infective. Brexit is specifically notable and damaging to people in the Southeast of the UK and London, where inhabitants have always been strongly anti-Brexit. New strains of the virus appear everywhere and continually. In the UK, a specifically performant detection system incidentally notes this new strain. The happening is not caused by this new strain but by mass hysteria in a region that happens to harbor this strain.

This would not be the first recent case of mass hysteria with an adverse effect on health. See chapter 'Pandemia or Global Hysteria?' for some examples (October 2019, at Starehe Girls Centre, Kenya; September 2018, Emirates Flight 203). The happening in the Southeast of the UK may just show that this kind of phenomenon is not bound to any single culture or circumstance. Moreover, stress makes people more unpredictably prone to suggestion.

Question: does this strain show to be more transmissible outside of the 'hysterical region'? If not, then this provides an additional pointer to a huge importance of 'stress' – as an immensely complex phenomenon – in the global COVID pandemic.

Simply COVID

Message to 'Two decades after' (today)

September 11, 2021

	Daily	Total
Cases worldwide	600.724	223.382.870
Deaths worldwide	9.772	4.608.917

Plus: many more deaths have already happened and are happening through COVID-related famine, worldwide.

The 'Minding Corona' reasoning, simply put, in 7 bullet points:

- Mind = body. There is no influence of something ephemeral upon something material. Change of mind = change of body. Please, wake up to this or stop reading.
- The placebo effect (and its counter-cousin, the nocebo effect) shows that health can be affected by sheer expectation-related suggestion in many domains to substantial degrees.
- Social nocebo (joint negative expectations by groups) is extensively investigated and shows to be potentially fatal.
- A lot of research shows the 'influence of mind' (see above) on immune-inflammatory (dys)function, which is heavily related to COVID morbidity and mortality.
- As a whirlpool-like phenomenon, mind-related and virus-related factors can draw COVID-patients increasingly down. Getting in or out of this whirlpool can mean a distinction between life or death.
- COVID vaccinations work, but in view of (very) flawed initial studies, we have no clue how big their placebo effect is — better

seen as a diminishment of nocebo (= getting out of the whirlpool).

- Personal and group-related instruments are available for scientific investigations and management. [see: "Proving and Using the Mind in COVID"] I cannot do so by myself. Please, help. At least, try to see it as helping yourself!

An App to Support

You may have read the whole book or just 'Minding COVID: a Different Story' and found out the broader why. In view of this, one may ask what can be done at the individual level. For this, an app is available containing mental exercises and supportive information. The present content of this app is for free forever for everyone. How it works: It doesn't. At least not

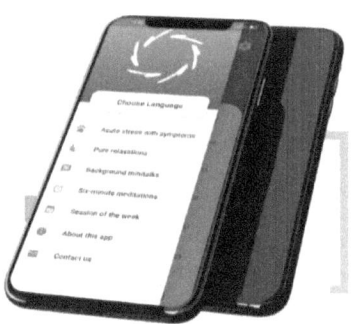

in the way of some medication, which it isn't. It would be mind-boggling to think or talk about it or use it that way. This said, you can see it as a key to the door that leads to your Inner Strength. I write these two words with capitals not because there is something supernatural involved. On the contrary, it is very natural: nature within you. In many situations, including COVID, this may diminish the negative strength of the whirlpool. This may be enough to either not get caught in it, or heighten the chance to get out of it with less damage. Theoretically, it may be life-saving. Of course, it needs to be said that as yet, no experimental research has been performed in this vein, due to a lack of resources.

So little with such huge consequences?

Well, it's relatively little, but please don't underestimate the know-how of years that has gone into the exercises as a whole and in detail. Also involved is clear ethics combining rationality and human depth. [see: "AURELIS USP: '100% Rationality, 100% Depth'"]. This combination is, within AURELIS, always of utmost importance. You may have confidence in this. It's all the way through.

So, with relatively little, a lot can be accomplished. But nothing magical. The app will not keep the virus out of your body. It will not have any direct impact whatsoever upon the virus. But it will have an impact on how your body-mind-unity reacts to the virus. That's at least already half of the story.

Imagine being present effectively somewhere outside of a whirlpool. You are quite near the whirlpool, but you don't see it for what it is. You see and fear the possible consequences. You know that something is there that can have a devastating effect upon you. It may even kill you. Of course, what you should avoid then is to step right into it. Without guidance, this may be precisely what many people do and what you also are at risk of doing. Your moves are crucial.

Imagine, unfortunately, getting into it and suffering the consequences.

Then imagine, with the proper guidance that this app can provide you, moving into the other direction. You are saved!

So, what is the difference?

In principle, not much in what you just did. You went one way or another. Yet, in consequence, the difference is immense.

Even if you are already within the whirlpool, not all is lost. Hopefully, excellent physicians will help you to get out of it. Besides that, this app can support you from a very different angle. It would be best if you used all the support you can get. One should not stand in the way of the other. it's crucial. It's your choice.

I hope you will make the right choice.

> You find the app as Aurelis in app stores. Or you can go to
> https://aurelis.org/aurelis-app
> On that same page, you find an intro video of the app.

Why the AURELIS app "cannot work against COVID"

Rest assured, there is much more to show that it can.
The AURELIS app is available in the app stores. You can find more information about it in the last appendix.

Apart from the blunt "This is not possible," or anything in that vein, I think of these arguments:

- COVID is a viral disease. Something purely mental cannot work.
- If the 'purely mental' – through using the app, for instance – worked, we would already know.
- I don't see how exactly this could be possible.
- The ephemeral mind cannot influence the physical body in any case.
- The mind can only make one feel better.
- This looks like a regression to magic.
- This would be something like telekinesis in which I don't believe.
- This lies outside of biomedical science.
- I don't encounter 'the mind' this way in my practice.
- The app is not experimentally proven to work against COVID.
- The entire world of medical science cannot be so wrong.
- It's impossible to just decide to become physically better.
- People cannot die through the influence of the mind.
- This is too simple to be effective.
- It is based on a weird hypothesis without circumstantial evidence.

However

There is more than enough answer to each of these arguments at other places in *Minding Corona* and the AURELIS-wiki. If you are a factual person, you may, for instance, want to read "Facts, Facts, Facts in Medicine."

If you can think of another argument for the list above, please let me know.

Otherwise, please take this free app seriously! Note that COVID is not mentioned on the app. 'Acute stress with symptoms' is relevant to many domains.

Afterword

The ravage that we have seen throughout many parts of the world in the last half year has taken us by surprise. What we will see in the twelve months to come will apparently also take many by surprise. It will be at least as bad and probably much worse than what has happened until now. We will see either an even more extended lockdown or even more dead and, one can say, wounded: people with long-lasting complications, about which not much is reported in the media. Most probably, it will be lockdown *and* way too many deaths.

That is: unless some wonder medication or procedure turns up. Super-vaccine? Super-selective immunomodulator? Taking the mind into proper consideration?

This book is the story of my journey into the latter. I have been traveling on this road much longer. Part of the journey lies in trying to understand the human mind from several viewpoints. When COVID struck, I was completely absorbed with what shows most of all how urgent is the need to understand ourselves in view of another part of this journey, oriented towards a future of Compassionate A.I. It is, after all, the same journey. The 'lesson of the virus' is our need to take ourselves seriously. As a species, we have created as well as destroyed many interesting things. Our future is now mainly dependent on our insight into who we are and what we will do with this knowledge.

I still think that every human being, as a total person, is immensely beautiful and interesting. However, in mere-ego, we tend to get stuck in an infinitesimal part of ourselves. In this part, we may think that we are in full conscious control of ourselves. We may think that nonconscious, subconceptual processing does not exist or is not relevant. Regarding the human mind, many people still act as medieval citizens who, looking at the sky at night, thought that the stars were stuck in a quintessence veil around the earth and that the earth — a flat disk — itself was all that matters in the universe. Meanwhile, we see the immense universe around us, but we still don't see the universe inside. Logically, this creates a lot of tension. Much of our technology helps us to do the things we do wrong more efficiently. The result, in many ways, creates more tension and stress.

Being busy with this for a long time, the new virus struck me as one that has found the niche of stressed-out organisms. Among other things, it soon became apparent that most of the sickness and death of the virus' victims came from an overreaction of the immune system. Mind — nervous system — immune system: The links are over-evident and, even so, only part of the relevant stuff that connects the mind to COVID. Scientifically too, we know so much about it. From the start on and even now, the lack of virus-related interest in this in the midst of a world ablaze is stunning.

However, after all — not really amazing to me — having just written extensively about the 'basic cognitive illusion.' That is: seeing *from* the deeper mind (universe inside) while not seeing the deeper mind itself. Even more, at the same time, I was finishing *Your Mind as Cure*, in which I delved into the importance of the deeper mind on health and healing. It's the basic tenet of my PhD-thesis, brought to the broader public. Reading this, one may see how omnipresent is this basic cognitive illusion, and how devastating to the health of many. One can look at it positively: how immense the possibilities are towards better health. I would add: and to a better future, period, as simple as that.

We are heading towards a world of A.I., in which our getting beyond our basic cognitive illusion will be the decisive factor between almost-heaven and almost-hell. This doesn't diminish the present viral urgency. Most interestingly, it shows that the same journey on which I stumbled is most crucial to both domains (and more).

So, I created the 'Aurelis-app.' It's not a complicated one by far. It's straightforward to use. Having read this book, you know dexamethasone (end of Chapter 6 and Chapter 11). You can look at the app as the 'dexamethasone of mind-related support.' It's ready-to-use, simple-to-use, efficient, cheap, and almost everywhere available. Differences are that it's safer and, well, more interesting. The real complexity lies in the autosuggestion-technology that I have been developing for 20 years. That's how I had no learning curve in applying it to the present situation.

You can also see the app as a key to the door to yourself. This key by itself does not 'do' anything, but you can use it to reach a space of utmost importance. You need to know how, but there is also support to this within the app itself. What may mostly stand in the way is the basic cognitive illusion. We need to get rid of that, most urgently of anything, as an individual, a society, and a species. If we don't, humanity is lost, not through the virus but the bi-bottleneck, as I have described in my A.I. book.

I am confident that we will not be able to do so by ourselves. Surprisingly, there's help around the corner. This help is A.I. itself, if developed and if it gets self-developing in a Compassionate way. We don't have to wait for this. We can build on it now, with present-day technology, used in innovative ways. I'm talking about an A.I.-coach that guides people to self-reflection, self-insight, and the diminishment of inner dissociation — a kind of power-turbo-Aurelis-app. The main challenge lies at the conceptual level. I have worked on this [see: "Lisa"] really hard specifically over 2019, but already from +/- 1993. Back then, I thought more positively about the future in many ways. Back now, bringing together the appropriate people, a first preliminary, yet already useful version would take a few months and at the cost of a fraction of what it will save purely economically. Just in time? No, not in view of the daily thousands of dead and wounded people around the world. Still, well before the main hammer will probably hit Europe and the US in the first months of 2021.

Today is 29 June 2020.

About the Author

Dr. Jean-Luc Mommaerts studied general and occupational medicine. He obtained degrees in Knowledge Systems and Hypnotherapy and is a Master of Cognitive Science and Artificial Intelligence. Jean-Luc worked as a physician for 12 years. At Kluwer Editorial, he was responsible for the development of a medical decision support system. At Language & Computing, he was responsible for a team of medical knowledge engineers. In 2014, he obtained a Ph.D. in medical science on the thesis "Subconceptual Processing in Medicine: From Body & Mind to Health & Healing." At present, apart from a COVID-intermezzo, his primary focus lies in developing a coaching chatbot, Lisa, based on subconceptual ('connectionist') principles.

Previous books

Dr. Jean-Luc Mommaerts is the author of *Your Mind as Cure*, in which he shows extensively and with much attention to science, yet in plain language, the importance of this book's title in many domains. In a few designated chapters and for everyone who wishes to delve into this, deeper levels of science are exposed in an accessible way. During the last few decades, it has become more and more apparent that the mind has a significant impact on health and healing. However, one needs to go way beyond mere 'positive thinking.' The conclusion is that human beings have much more inner strength available than is generally thought. Nobody can give you that strength as if it were some medication, but everybody can attain it and receive support towards doing so.

In *The Journey Towards Compassionate A.I.*, Dr. Mommaerts brings together present-day scientific insights about meaningfulness, information, intelligence, and consciousness, demonstrating that there is no 'magic' involved. This book also indicates their importance to Compassion. Finally, it shows the proximity of *real* artificial intelligence and, shortly afterward, artificial consciousness, thereby 'soon enough' making Compassionate A.I. personally crucial for everyone and even an existential issue for humanity. *The Journey* is a book for anyone who cares about the future in which super-A.I. will play the dominant role. Soon enough, that future will become the present. We already see substantial negative consequences: mass manipulations in social media, A.I.-driven autonomous drones as weapons of mass destruction, etc. Yet the current surge in 'so-called A.I.' is still the preliminary phase. Meanwhile, a lot is going on in the domain of cognitive neuroscience. Researchers gain real insights into concepts that lie close to our hearts – and brains. But these researchers are mainly working in their silos. The author unifies the 'depths of human being' with a rational take on "who we are, what A.I. can become, and why it matters."

Books by Dr. Jean-Luc Mommaerts

- The Journey Towards Compassionate A.I.
- Your Mind as Cure
- Minding Corona
- Read&Do: Open leadership
- Read&Do: Stressional Intelligence
- Read&Do: Getting Slim
- Read&Do: Chronic Pain Relief
- Read&Do: Burnout Prevention
- Read&Do: Open Mindfulness
- Read&Do: Depression Relief
- Read&Do: Quit Smoking
- Read&Do: Deep Motivation
- Sticky Thoughts
- Poems from a Parallel World

AURELIS Mission

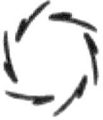

AURELIS = tapping into the possibilities that arise from optimal communication with the deeper self (the 'nonconscious'), in the language of and deep respect for the deeper self. The goal is to intensely invite the total person to organic growth so that change in the right direction acquires a deep spontaneity. As a result, the individual comes to live in a different way, namely from within and thus transcending the ego, in greater harmony with himself and the world. The dissociation between consciousness and the nonconscious diminishes. The power of the nonconscious is largely released to be used for consciously chosen goals. The total person acts as a unity and realizes in a powerful way who he really is and, on closer inspection, always has been. AURELIS is an extension of positive thinking but goes much further. AURELIS starts where positive thinking ends: at the real limits of the deeper self. The movement of AURELIS is the movement of the flower bud that opens spontaneously into a beautiful flower in the light of the sun. Keywords are: openness, deep attention, total non-aggression, truth, rationality and feeling, the total person, organic growth.

www.aurelis.org